Feasting on Emotions

The Psychology of Binge Eating

by

Sara Parkes

Table of Contents

Introduction

Embarking on a journey towards understanding oneself can be both challenging and profound; when dealing with binge eating disorder (BED), it's an imperative exploration. This book serves as a beacon for those who suspect they might grapple with the silent thralls of BED, aiming to shed light on identifying the condition, uncovering its underlying causes, and navigating through the multitude of treatment options available. BED is not merely a disruption of eating patterns but a complex interplay of psychological, physiological, and societal factors which deeply influence an individual's well-being (American Psychiatric Association, 2013). In this moment, pause and consider the courage it takes to explore such a deeply personal issue and let this book be a testament to that bravery. The subsequent chapters do not merely outline clinical facts and treatments but offer a keen understanding and guidance on embarking upon a transformative path to not just recovery but sustainable self-empowerment and health.

Chapter 1:
Understanding Binge Eating Disorder (BED)

As we delve into the complexities of Binge Eating Disorder (BED), we uncover a condition that's both deeply personal and widely misunderstood. BED isn't just about indulging to excess; it's a recognized psychiatric disorder defined by recurrent episodes of eating large quantities of food, a feeling of loss of control during the binge, experiencing shame or guilt afterwards, and not regularly using unhealthy compensatory measures to counter the binge eating (American Psychiatric Association, 2013). This disorder exists on a spectrum with various eating disorders, bearing unique characteristics that distinguish it from occasional overeating or other disordered eating behaviors. The nuances of BED go beyond the act of eating, mirroring complexities within the human psyche and embodying a nexus where the brain, behavior, and societal influences converge.

Defining BED

Binge Eating Disorder, commonly known by the acronym BED, is a complex and serious condition characterized by recurring episodes of eating large quantities of food, often quickly and to the point of discomfort. These episodes are usually marked by a feeling of loss of control, followed by significant distress or guilt. BED stands as the most common eating disorder in the United States, affecting millions across different ages and backgrounds. It transcends the mere action of overeating, engulfing one's emotional and psychological spheres, making it pivotal to discern its essence beyond the plate.

To truly grasp the gravity and nuances of BED, it's essential to acknowledge its inclusion in the Diagnostic and Statistical Manual of Mental Disorders, Fifth Edition (DSM-5). This incorporation not only validated the struggles of many but also laid down specific criteria for diagnosis (American Psychiatric Association, 2013). Unlike other eating disorders, BED does not regularly involve compensatory behaviors like purging, fasting, or excessive exercise. Such detail is fundamentally significant because BED is not about the food itself; it's about the struggle within, where food becomes a coping mechanism for underlying issues, often obscured by societal stigma and misconceptions.

The courage to confront BED head-on begins with understanding, empathy, and scientific scrutiny. Acknowledging BED's real impact is a pivotal step in the journey of healing. By defining this disorder, we're not merely setting diagnostic boundaries; we're uncovering the layers of personal pain, societal pressures, and biological underpinnings that contribute to its manifestation. It's a journey that requires a compassionate yet analytical approach, one that doesn't merely dwell at the surface but dives deep into the torrents of one's inner workings to emerge with insight and hope for recovery (Kessler et al., 2013).

The Spectrum of Eating Disorders

As we delve deeper into the examination of Binge Eating Disorder (BED), it's crucial to understand its placement within the spectrum of eating disorders. While BED is distinguished by recurrent episodes of eating large quantities of food, often rapidly and to the point of discomfort, it's one of multiple eating disorders recognized by health professionals. This spectrum encompasses conditions such as Anorexia Nervosa, Bulimia Nervosa, and Other Specified Feeding or Eating Disorders (OSFED), each varied in their manifestations but united by a central disturbance in eating behavior and an excessive preoccupation with body weight or shape (American Psychiatric Association, 2013).

Eating disorders are complex mental health conditions not chosen by those who suffer from them, but rather are serious illnesses with potentially life-threatening conditions. These disorders often coexist with other psychiatric disorders such as depression, anxiety, and substance abuse, complicating the individual's emotional canvas, which must be navigated with great care (Ulfvebrand et al., 2015).

In comprehending the spectrum, one must also recognize the uniqueness of each disorder. Anorexia Nervosa is characterized primarily by self-starvation and excessive weight loss, while Bulimia Nervosa includes a cycle of binge eating followed by compensatory behaviors such as vomiting or excessive exercise. BED, on the other hand, lacks these compensatory behaviors. However, individuals with BED often experience feelings of shame, guilt, and loss of control over their eating, similar to those with Bulimia Nervosa (Kessler et al., 2013).

Between these well-defined conditions are the nuances and variations represented by OSFED. This categorization includes those who do not meet the complete criteria for Anorexia or Bulimia but still exhibit significant disordered eating behaviors. For instance, an individual might experience episodes of binge eating without the regular use of compensating mechanisms as in Bulimia, which could be classified as OSFED (American Psychiatric Association, 2013).

The importance of understanding this spectrum is multifaceted. Recognizing the different manifestations can be important for identifying BED; each disorder requires a tailored approach to treatment. While this section focuses on BED, it's crucial to differentiate it from its counterparts as such differentiations inform both diagnostics and intervention strategies. The variations across the spectrum mean that a one-size-fits-all approach is ineffective. Interventions must be as unique as the individual and their specific challenges with eating and body image.

This spectrum also underlines the potential for progression or transition between disorders. It's not uncommon for sufferers to move from one eating disorder into another over time, which makes early and accurate diagnosis all the more essential (Treasure et al., 2015). Understanding the full spectrum can aid in prevention, enabling sufferers and care providers to spot early warning signs before an individual transitions from disordered eating behaviors to a full-blown eating disorder.

For those grappling with BED or any eating disorder, the path to recovery often feels daunting. Realizing that BED is but one facet of a wider array of eating disorders can provide a context for understanding personal experiences. It is part of a complex but navigable map of mental health conditions. Effective treatment necessitates recognizing where one is on this spectrum and approaching recovery with a comprehensive, evidence-based strategy.

It must be emphasized that while the conditions across the spectrum share certain underlying similarities, such as issues with self-esteem and body image, the divergences are equally significant. As we move forward into exploring ways to identify and treat BED, the core principle remains clear: a deep, empathetic understanding of the spectrum is indispensable for anyone on the journey toward healing and recovery.

As the discussion progresses, the focus will remain steadfast on BED, yet always within the broader landscape of eating disorders. This perspective allows individuals to contextualize their experiences while receiving the specialized care that their particular condition demands.

BED vs. Other Eating Behaviors

Understanding the distinction between Binge Eating Disorder (BED) and other eating behaviors is crucial to identifying and addressing the underlying causes of this condition. While BED shares certain characteristics with other disordered eating patterns, such as overeating, emotional eating, and other specified feeding or eating disorders (OSFED), there are distinct differences that must be emphasized to provide appropriate interventions and support.

Overeating is a behavior that many individuals may experience from time to time, often as a normal response to situational cues such as social gatherings or exceptionally palatable food. Unlike overeating, BED is characterized by recurrent episodes of consuming unusually large amounts of food in a specific time frame, accompanied by a sense of lack of control and significant emotional distress. These episodes occur at least once a week for three months, a frequency not typically seen in general overeating behaviors (American Psychiatric Association, 2013). Furthermore, emotional eating – although it may lead to overeating – does not always result in the loss of control and is not necessarily a precursor to BED.

Additionally, BED is set apart from other eating disorders like anorexia nervosa and bulimia nervosa, by the absence of consistent compensatory behaviors such as purging, fasting, or excessive exercise. OSFED, which may manifest with a variety of symptoms that do not neatly fit into the criteria of other eating disorders, can sometimes be confused with BED. However, BED is a diagnostic category in its own right, characterized by unique behavioral, emotional, and cognitive patterns (Kessler et al., 2013). Understanding these distinctions is paramount for healthcare professionals to make an accurate diagnosis and to develop targeted and effective treatment interventions, steering individuals towards a path of recovery that acknowledges the complexity and individuality of their experiences with food.

Chapter 2:
How to Identify BED

As we continue to unravel the complexities of Binge Eating Disorder (BED), it's crucial to begin with the foundational step of identifying if you are grappling with this conundrum. The task at hand isn't merely to list symptoms, but to engage with them, to understand the subtleties of your eating patterns and emotional responses with a keen, introspective eye. Picture those days when food becomes a hidden solace, or when eating is no longer attached to hunger but to a ravenous emotional void; these are the flickers that might suggest the presence of BED (American Psychological Association [APA], 2013). It isn't just about what you eat, but the why and the how - the secretive binges, the feeling of loss of control, and the subsequent waves of guilt and shame. Self-assessment tools are readily available to bridge the gap between silent struggles and vocalizing your battles, but they're simply the scouts ahead of the cavalry, which, in this case, are trained professionals who can confirm a diagnosis and guide you on the path to reclaiming control. Identifying BED is akin to sketching a map of an unfamiliar territory—it starts with a few lines, often obscured and shaky, but with each honest acknowledgment and professional insight, the picture becomes clearer, nudging you towards the road to recovery and empowerment.

Recognizing the Symptoms of Binge Eating Disorder (BED) is a pivotal step towards understanding and embracing the journey to recovery. The impediments we face on the path to wellness often stem from our inability to identify the subtle yet persistent signs that something within us cries out for attention and care. It's often a clandestine struggle, marked by episodes of consuming large quantities of food within a short time frame, feelings of distress or loss of control during these episodes, and an absence of compensatory behaviors like those present in bulimia nervosa (American Psychiatric Association, 2013).

Symptoms of BED can manifest as eating much more rapidly than normal, and eating until uncomfortably full. It's not uncommon to eat large amounts of food when not feeling physically hungry or to eat alone due to embarrassment by how much one is consuming. After such binges, one may experience overwhelming guilt, disgust, or shame. Yet, it's this very acknowledgment of distress that can act as a blaring siren, urging us to seek transformation.

Understanding that binge eating often occurs in secrecy is essential. This symptom not only exacerbates the shame associated with BED but also serves as a barrier to seeking help. The recurring nature of binge eating, typically at least once a week for three months, is a clinical criterion that distinguishes occasional overeating from a diagnosable disorder. This temporal pattern can serve as a clear signal that intervention might be necessary, a song of hope on the horizon that with the right help, change is possible.

Another aspect of recognizing BED symptoms is realizing the difference between emotional hunger and physical hunger. Emotional hunger is an urgent need to consume food in response to feelings other than hunger, such as stress or sadness, which leads to more rapid eating without physical cues of hunger. Contrarily, physical hunger develops gradually and can be satisfied with a variety of foods. Distinguishing between the two types of hunger can empower someone with BED to understand their eating patterns and recognize the triggers that drive their behavior.

In the grand scheme of symptoms, it's paramount to remember that while certain signs can point to BED, they are not markers of failure or character flaws. They are signals, signposts on the road to recovery beckoning us forward. It's through this lens of self-compassion and determination that we can grasp the full scope of BED and embark on a journey not defined by our eating habits but by the strength of our spirit to overcome and thrive.

Self-Assessment Tools form a pivotal chapter in your journey towards understanding Binge Eating Disorder (BED). As we unpack the mechanisms behind BED's pervasive grip, we alight upon a powerful step: introspection facilitated by self-assessment. These tools are not diagnostic instruments, but they can be revealing indicators of patterns and behaviors often associated with BED (Smith et al., 2020). It's vital to approach these assessments with an open mind, understanding that self-examination is both a brave and necessary stride towards healing.

One of the most accessible forms of self-assessment is the self-report questionnaire. Typically, these questionnaires include a series of statements about eating habits, emotional state, and body image. You respond based on your experiences, which provides immediate insight into your behaviors and emotions surrounding food. These questionnaires often draw from established clinical scales and offer a quantified glimpse into the potential severity of binge eating symptoms. This can serve as compelling preliminary evidence that one's relationship with food may require a more in-depth evaluation.

Another tool is the food diary, a self-monitored record of eating behaviors. By tracking what, when, and how much you eat, alongside the emotions and context of each episode, you gather concrete data about your eating patterns. This tool can unearth triggers for binge eating, highlight unhealthy patterns, and reveal emotional connections to food consumption, making it an invaluable resource in the self-assessment arsenal (Leahy et al., 2017).

Reflection prompts and introspective guides also play a crucial role in self-assessment. These tools encourage you to delve deeper into your thoughts and feelings, uncovering the psychological substrates that contribute to binge eating behaviors. They work to peel back the layers, fostering a deeper understanding of the emotional and cognitive drivers that propel you towards binge eating. This nurtures a profound self-awareness, vital for targeted treatment and therapeutic intervention.

It's crucial to note that while these tools offer a window into your relationship with food, they are not substitutes for professional evaluation. They are the preliminary steps that arm you with valuable insights, which when shared with a healthcare professional, can streamline the diagnostic process and tailor the treatment plan to your specific needs. To echo the sentiment of this book's mission, self-awareness is the beacon that lights the path to discovering the underlying causes of BED and the bespoke treatments that await beyond (Smith et al., 2020).

When to Seek Professional Help

Understanding when to seek professional assistance for Binge Eating Disorder (BED) is pivotal in the journey to recovery and well-being. While self-assessment tools and recognition of symptoms are crucial first steps, distinguishing when those symptoms signal the need for professional help is sometimes challenging. Individuals struggling with frequent episodes of eating unusually large amounts of food, feeling a lack of control during these episodes, and experiencing distress or impairment due to their eating behavior may be facing a serious health condition that necessitates professional insight (Smith et al., 2021).

The transition from occasional overeating to what could be a diagnosable case of BED often involves a complex mix of psychological, physiological, and behavioral factors. It is important to consult with a healthcare provider when there is a persistent pattern of binge eating, which can manifest through rapid eating until uncomfortably full, eating large amounts when not hungry, and feeling self-disgust or guilt post-binge. These signs underscore the importance of taking the leap from self-help attempts to seeking trained professionals who can offer a holistic approach to treatment.

Moreover, should the episodes of binge eating lead to marked distress, including anxiety, depression, or significant health concerns such as weight fluctuations, gastrointestinal issues, or metabolic abnormalities, it's time to engage with healthcare practitioners. Importantly, consulting professionals becomes urgent if binge eating behaviors are co-occurring with other mental health concerns, such as mood disorders or substance abuse, as these complexities often require specialized interventions.

Professional help can be sought in various forms, including but not limited to, physicians, psychologists, or registered dietitians specialized in eating disorders. These experts not only diagnose and treat BED but can help individuals understand and tackle the underlying causes of their eating patterns, whether they be emotional triggers, stress, or trauma. Through tailored treatment plans, which may include therapy, medication, or nutritional counseling, individuals find themselves supported in a structured pathway towards sustained recovery and well-being.

Overall, when self-directed efforts to manage binge eating do not yield the desired progress, or when the severity of the disorder escalates, it becomes imperative to reach out for professional help. Attaining a balanced relationship with food and overcoming the triggers of BED is often a collaborative effort; professionals offer the necessary guidance for those looking to reclaim control and lead a healthier life both mentally and physically. As individuals consider their next steps, they should acknowledge that reaching out signifies strength and commitment to their health and should be regarded as a positive and proactive approach on the path to recovery.

Chapter 3:
Diagnosis of BED

Having unpacked the ways to discern the presence of Binge Eating Disorder (BED), we pivot now to the crucial fulcrum of the journey: its formal diagnosis. A mosaic of intricate patterns, BED requires a diagnostician's eye to illuminate its contours, an undertaking that wields the tools of methodical analysis and empathetic understanding. The professional evaluation process is a meticulous venture, an alchemy of medical diagnostics that adhere strictly to established criteria in manuals such as the DSM-5. As we explore the clinical pathways that lead to a BED diagnosis, we also recognize that acceptance of the diagnosis itself is a threshold many hesitate to cross due to stigma and misconceptions. By recognizing the legitimacy of BED as a diagnosable condition, we empower individuals to step through shame's shadows into the clarity of acknowledgment and, subsequently, towards healing. This chapter navigates the reader through the intricacies of the medical, psychological, and societal dimensions that converge in the diagnosis of BED, providing clarity on a cornerstone of the healing journey.

The Professional Evaluation Process

In the expanse of our exploration into Binge Eating Disorder (BED), we've educated ourselves about its gnarly roots and multifaceted expressions. We know it's there, but how exactly is BED identified in a clinical setting? That's where the professional evaluation process becomes our compass in the murky waters of diagnosis. It's a crucial juncture, where individuals are sculpted from question marks into a clear path toward healing and understanding.

The professional evaluation for BED is multilayered and nothing short of meticulous. Qualified health care providers—be it psychologists, psychiatrists, or general health practitioners—use a blend of diagnostic criteria, such as those found in the Diagnostic and Statistical Manual of Mental Disorders, alongside their clinical experience. The initial evaluation delves into one's eating habits, psychological wellbeing, and physical health condition. The professional discerns patterns, frequency, and severity of binge eating episodes, and they're equally attentive to concurrent symptoms, such as depression, anxiety, or body dysmorphia, which often interlace with BED.

But these sessions go beyond ticking boxes of symptoms. The therapeutic embrace of evaluation is about forging trust, understanding the person's story, and the factors that fuel their behavior. During this liaison, empirical evidence is woven with personal narratives. This is the dance of science and lived experience, performed in the service of reaching an accurate diagnosis. Listening becomes a tool just as invaluable as any psychological assessment.

Confronting the possibility of BED necessitates a series of follow-up evaluations. Recovery isn't binary; it ebbs and flows with life's unpredictable tides. Hence, professionals keep a weather eye on progress, setbacks, and evolution in symptoms. Collaboratively, with their clients, they navigate the shapeshifting journey of BED, ensuring that a diagnosis morphs into a tailored roadmap for treatment and recovery. This process is not set in stone—it adapts, flexes, and matures as it mirrors the individual's unique recovery trek.

To articulate the profound tapestry of this condition, and to ultimately transcend its grip, an individual must walk through the pivotal gateway of professional evaluation. It's here that clarity and treatment tether, and where the initial threads of recovery are woven. Embedding oneself in this process is an act of bravery—and the vital first step in reclaiming autonomy over one's health and well-being.

Medical Diagnostics and Criteria Essence lies in the truth we face, not the myths we chase. When investigating the abyss of Binge Eating Disorder (BED), a steadfast beacon is the medical diagnostic framework. Its importance cannot be overstated in identifying the condition, distinguishing it from others, and paving the way for effective intervention. The journey towards understanding and identifying BED is incomplete without discussing the cornerstone that defines its medical diagnosis and criteria.

Through the lens of an unsung detective, we embark on the meticulous process of diagnosis. It's not an overstatement to say that thorough clinical evaluation is the backbone of managing BED. Physicians and mental health professionals employ established criteria, notably from the Diagnostic and Statistical Manual of Mental Disorders, Fifth Edition (DSM-5), to illuminate the path toward precise identification of BED. The DSM-5 insists upon recurrent episodes of binge eating characterized by two cardinal elements: eating an objectively large amount of food within a discrete time frame and a sense of lack of control during these episodes.

The diagnostic criteria elaborate further, specifying that binge-eating episodes are accompanied by three or more symptoms, such as eating much more rapidly than normal, eating until uncomfortably full, or eating large amounts of food when not physically hungry. Another key aspect of the diagnostic criteria stresses that significant distress is present regarding binge eating and that this behavior occurs at least once a week for three months. One must distinguish BED from bulimia nervosa, ensuring the absence of recurrent compensatory behaviors like purging.

It's not an overreach to say that a physical exam and comprehensive medical history are pivotal. They stand as reliable pillars, holding up the weight of differential diagnosis. Physicians look to exclude medical conditions that could mimic binge-eating symptoms, such as Prader-Willi syndrome, a genetic disorder with an insatiable appetite as a hallmark (Goldstone et al., 2018). Lab tests and screenings mitigate the risk of attributing symptoms to BED that actually signal other concerns, like thyroid disorders or hormone imbalances influencing appetite.

The importance of diagnostic precision is akin to navigating a complex labyrinth with a map - it provides clear direction in a maze of uncertainty. This process gives patients and professionals alike the means to measure the efficacy of treatments and gauge recovery progress. Notwithstanding the value of a professional diagnosis, self-assessment tools serve as an initial checkpoint for those pondering whether they might be contending with BED. They're the flashlight in the dark, before comprehensive situational light is shed by a healthcare provider's full-fledged evaluation.

In a world where early detection can influence the entire trajectory of a disorder, understanding and utilizing these criteria becomes not just a matter of academic interest, but a vital, life-altering tool. Key to this endeavor is overcoming stigma, which often discourages sufferers from seeking help. The medical community's empathetic approach to discussing BED criteria can become a balm, soothing the open wound of shame that prevents many from stepping forward.

Let's remember that the criterion established by medical professionals is not meant to label or stigmatize but to clarify and guide. Embracing this diagnostic framework allows us to confront the lurking shadows of BED head-on. Once diagnosed, the individual has, in essence, taken the first step out of the shadows and into the light of potential recovery.

Lest we believe the journey ends there, it is merely the starting point. The path follows through with appropriate treatment modalities such as medication, therapy, and nutritional support, each selected based on the individual's unique presentation of BED, and all underpinned by the specific criteria met in the diagnosis. Moreover, recognizing the diagnostic criteria aids in the ongoing development of more nuanced and personalized therapeutic interventions.

Thus, the quest toward managing BED begins with the demystification of its symptoms through medical diagnostics and criteria. This knowledge becomes the mighty sword with which individuals and healthcare providers can battle the dragon of BED, not in a mythical land but in the tangible reality of affective and evidence-based strategies.

Overcoming Stigma and Accepting Diagnosis

Building on our understanding of Binge Eating Disorder (BED) and its professional evaluation, we now face one of the most formidable barriers in the journey towards healing: overcoming the stigma and arriving at a place of acceptance. Acceptance is not merely about acknowledging a diagnosis; it's about welcoming this truth into our lives and allowing it to coexist with our identities without shame or self-reproach.

The stigma surrounding BED, much like other mental health disorders, is rooted in a lack of knowledge and an abundance of misconceptions. Individuals may worry that they will be labeled as lacking willpower or discipline. The echoes of societal judgments whisper that it's simply a matter of eating less and moving more. These pervasive attitudes contribute to feelings of shame and isolation.

However, acceptance starts with understanding that BED is not a reflection of character, but rather a complex disorder that intertwines biology, psychology, and social factors. Recognizing that the condition is a legitimate medical issue requiring professional assistance can be an empowering step. Accepting a diagnosis means stepping onto a path of self-compassion, which is essential for recovery.

A key step in fighting stigma is education, both personal and communal. Arming oneself with knowledge about the disorder transforms the internal narrative from one of blame to one of advocacy. Education fosters empathy, for oneself and from others, carving a path through the thicket of stigma.

Moreover, connecting with others who are struggling with the same issues can provide a robust support system that contradicts feelings of solitude and alienation. Peer support groups and online forums reinforce the narrative that no one is alone in this fight. Here, the shared experiences of struggle and triumph serve as the collective power that marginalizes the effects of stigma.

Educating friends and family is an additional layer in creating a bedrock of support. When loved ones understand the challenges of BED, they can be indispensable allies. They cease to be part of the external pressure, instead becoming key components of the recovery process, a fortress against the tide of stigma.

Personal growth and identity reformation are intertwined with acceptance. The diagnosis of BED does not encapsulate one's being— it is merely a component. Redefining oneself beyond the disorder is vital, affirming that personhood is composed of multifaceted experiences and attributes, only one of which is battling with BED.

The role of healthcare professionals in this process should not be understated. When a diagnosis is delivered with empathy, clarity, and devoid of judgment, it sets a precedent for how individuals should treat themselves. Providers must lead by example in casting aside bias and conveying respect.

Confronting internalized stigma is similarly crucial. The harshest critic can often be oneself. Through therapeutic modalities, such as Cognitive-Behavioral Therapy (CBT), individuals learn to challenge and modify negative beliefs about themselves and the disorder, thereby fostering a more supportive internal dialogue.

Accepting a diagnosis does not mean resigning to it. It means mobilizing oneself for the journey ahead. It entails acknowledging the reality while simultaneously advocating for personal health and well-being. It is a declaration that one is ready to engage with treatment and pave the way for recovery.

As in any significant life alteration, the passage to acceptance is also about reshaping one's narrative. The stories we tell ourselves matter, and rewriting the internal script from one of failure to one of brave confrontation and proactive management changes how we approach each day, affecting our mindset and actions.

Furthermore, developing a sense of agency is a potent antidote to stigma. Realizing that there are steps one can take, treatments to follow, and changes that can be made puts the power back into the hands of the individual. This sense of control is a formidable tool in dismantling the shackles of stigma.

To encapsulate, the battle against BED and societal stigma is multifaceted. It requires resilience to overcome external prejudices, but more importantly, it demands courage to change the internal dialogue and embrace the diagnosis. The act of acceptance is not the end of the journey, but rather a bold step forward in the continuum of recovery and empowerment.

Chapter 4:
Psychological Implications and Causes of BED

Peeling back the layers of Binge Eating Disorder (BED) reveals a convoluted range of emotional triggers and psychological underpinnings. Every instance of loss of control in eating is not merely an isolated event; it's a symptom of deeper, often hidden emotional turmoil and mental distress. It is within this chapter that we unravel these complex psychological threads. Research identifies that BED may stem from a discord between the individual's environment and psychological state, often fueled by critical incidents, persistent stress, or unresolved trauma. The intricacies of the brain's reward system, underscored by neuroscientific studies, also play a prominent role in the emergence and perpetuation of binge eating behaviors. The intertwining of neurobiology with emotional experiences creates a potent cocktail predisposing individuals to turn to food as a source of ephemeral solace. Understanding these factors is not only critical to recognizing the disorder but also empowering for those affected.

Emotional Triggers and Roots

Unearthing the emotional triggers and underlying roots of Binge Eating Disorder (BED) is akin to detective work, where patterns play the culprit, and emotional responses act as clues. At this juncture, one must recognize the multifaceted nature of BED, which not only includes physiological elements but also deep-seated emotional and psychological factors. It's crucial to understand that emotional triggers can engender powerful urges to binge eat, serving as a coping mechanism for adverse feelings and experiences.

The roots of these triggers are often buried in past traumas or unresolved psychological issues. Childhood experiences, such as criticism regarding weight or eating habits, can germinate into triggers in adulthood. Similarly, incidents of abuse, neglect, or significant loss can profoundly influence one's relationship with food. The role of such emotional catalysts cannot be underestimated, as they frequently lead individuals to seek solace in the temporary comfort of binge eating.

Moreover, chronic stress or an inability to express emotions healthily can fortify the cycle of BED. Day-to-day pressures, when not managed effectively, can accumulate and express themselves through disordered eating behaviors. The consumption of food in large quantities then momentarily masks feelings like stress, sadness, or anxiety. It's imperative to acknowledge that these short-term reprieves through food often exacerbate the very emotions they are intended to obscure.

Furthermore, social factors also play a pivotal role. The critical gaze of our aesthetically driven culture can foster feelings of inadequacy, often triggering disordered eating patterns in an effort to conform to societal expectations. Social isolation, too, can ignite the spark of binge eating, as the need for emotional connection and belonging remains unmet. The consequential feelings of loneliness and despair frequently convert into triggers for an individual with BED.

What becomes evident is the interplay between emotional triggers and their roots—an intricate network of personal history, daily interactions, and internal struggles. Being attuned to the causes of one's emotions is the first step towards disentangling oneself from the snare of BED. A profound understanding of this relationship facilitates the development of strategies aimed at mitigating these triggers and creating healthier coping mechanisms.

Effective intervention involves not just the cessation of binge eating episodes, but more importantly, an exploration into the emotional landscape where these triggers germinate. As those with BED seek to navigate through this terrain, self-reflection is paramount. Journaling, meditative practices, and therapies such as Cognitive-Behavioral Therapy (CBT) offer substantial aid in recognizing and managing these emotional triggers.

While this exploration can be confronting, it's also laced with the opportunity for radical transformation. As one interrogates the confluence of past pain and present challenges, the emergence of self-compassion becomes key. It is through a compassionate self-encounter that individuals learn to replace the ephemeral solace of binge eating with long-term, nurturing alternatives.

Finally, seeking the support of a mental health professional can serve as a cornerstone for unraveling the web of emotional triggers. The guidance of a therapist can illuminate the path towards healing, making the journey less daunting and more structured. The therapist's role encompasses aiding individuals in identifying triggers, unpacking the emotional intricacies, and building resilience against future triggers.

The Brain and Binge Eating

As we deepen our understanding of Binge Eating Disorder (BED), it's imperative to consider the multifaceted role of the brain. The brain is the command center, intricately involved in hunger cues, cravings, and emotional responses—all elements at play in binge eating. But what happens in the complex labyrinth of neural pathways to fuel such behaviors?

Investigations into the neural correlates of BED have shed light on the hyperactivation of the reward systems during food consumption (Balodis et al., 2013). In a neurobiological dance, the brain's dopamine pathways—typically signaling pleasure and reward—fire off intensely in response to food stimuli. This chemical rush can mimic those found in substance use disorders, clarifying why food can become such an addictive source. For those with BED, these neural fireworks can override the normal satiety signals, leading to continued eating despite physical fullness.

Yet, it's not just pure neuroscience at play here; emotions have their script in the narrative of binge eating. The amygdala, a brain region associated with emotional processing, also seems to work overtime when individuals with BED confront food, especially food associated with comfort or stress relief. This heightened emotional connectivity with food suggests that treatments targeting emotional regulation could be key in managing BED. It also highlights the importance of therapies that encompass mindfulness and cognitive restructuring, aiming to rewrite the emotional coding linked to eating behaviors.

Additionally, acknowledgment of the prefrontal cortex—the brain's decision-making hub—matters profoundly. In those struggling with BED, the prefrontal cortex often shows diminished activity, pointing towards a compromised ability to exert self-control and make reasoned choices regarding food intake. This insight into the neurological underpinnings of BED emphasizes why strategies leaning on sheer willpower often falter. Instead, therapeutic interventions need to focus on strengthening cognitive control and developing healthier coping mechanisms.

In summary, the brain's circuitry doesn't merely act as a backdrop; it is integral to the unfolding story of binge eating. Understanding these neural mechanisms isn't an academic exercise—it's a crucial step towards tailored, effective interventions. It's about harnessing the power of the brain's plasticity to retrain and build new pathways, forge better habits, and ultimately, regain control. Knowing the science is a beacon of hope; it assures that with the right strategies, recovery isn't just a possibility—it's within reach.

The Role of Stress and Trauma

Recognizing the profound impact of stress and trauma on individuals with Binge Eating Disorder (BED) is pivotal in understanding the full spectrum of this condition. Our journey through this exploration uncovers not just the superficial layers of eating habits but reaches into the deep, often unspoken realm of psychological distress.

The human response to stress is a tale as old as time, a complex symphony orchestrated by the brain under duress. In the context of BED, stress can act as both a precursor and perpetuator of binge eating episodes. It triggers a chain reaction, igniting the brain's reward centers and seeking solace where it can most immediately be found: food. Comfort eating is a well-documented phenomenon, a temporary haven from stress, albeit one with long-term consequences.

Trauma, whether physical or emotional, leaves indelible marks upon the psyche, often altering one's relationship with food and eating. Traumatic events can reshape the brain's wiring, priming individuals for psychological conditions like BED. The storage of traumatic memories, interwoven into the fabric of one's daily life, can repeatedly trigger stress responses that lead to binges. This act of eating serves as an attempt to dissociate from the pain, a maladaptive coping mechanism to blunt the sharp edges of trauma.

In considering the role of stress and trauma, we see their fingerprints in the narratives of many who struggle with BED. A stressful job, turbulent relationships, or a history of abuse can all act as kindling for the fire of binge eating behaviors. The immediacy of the stress-eating cycle is a trap that ensnares without prejudice, leaving in its wake a feeling of loss of control—an ironic predicament as the initial instinct was to regain a sense of command over one's emotional strife.

Unpacking the science behind stress and its physiological components opens a window into the mechanisms at play. The adrenal glands excrete cortisol during stress, a hormone that, in constant supply, can drive the compulsion to reach for high-calorie, sugary, and fatty foods (Tomiyama, 2019). This hormonal tide pushes one towards eating as a form of self-medication, a reprieve from the storm of hormonal fluctuations.

However, the aftermath of binge eating as a stress response is often a maelstrom of guilt, shame, and further stress—a vicious cycle where eating to relieve stress breeds more stress, which in turn feeds the cycle of binge eating. Acknowledging this pattern is the first step in breaking its chains.

Addressing trauma in the context of BED is delicate, requiring a nuanced approach attentive to individual experiences. Trauma-informed care is gaining recognition as a fundamental aspect of effective BED treatment, recognizing that many patients come with histories of trauma that impact their eating behaviors (Smith et al., 2020). This understanding shifts the paradigm from one of mere behavior modification to one that heals underlying wounds.

The therapeutic landscape for those grappling with stress-related binge eating is rich with possibility. Cognitive-behavioral therapy (CBT) arms individuals with the tools to reframe their relationship with food and build resilience against stress. Mindfulness practices cultivate a presence that buffers against the impulsivity of binge eating. Eye Movement Desensitization and Reprocessing (EMDR) therapy specifically targets traumatic memories, potentially unlocking a path to recovery for those whose BED is interlaced with past traumas.

Exploring the impact of adverse childhood experiences (ACEs) on eating behaviors has shed light on the roots of BED. ACEs, particularly those related to emotional and physical neglect, have been linked with a higher prevalence of eating disorders including BED. Unveiling these experiences and addressing the resultant emotional turmoil is a crucial element in the healing journey.

The intertwining of stress, trauma, and BED reveals the centrality of emotional well-being in addressing this disorder. The compulsion to eat is not merely a physical one but a signal highlighting deeper distress. Providing holistic care that encompasses physical, emotional, and psychological support is vital.

Encouragement, therefore, must be offered not only in embracing external treatment modalities but also in fostering inner resilience. This resilience emerges from an understanding of one's stressors, a reworking of one's responses to them, and the gradual building up of healthier coping strategies that step beyond the immediate gratification of food.

Moreover, societal pressures and stressors can't be ignored as contributing factors to BED. The relentless pursuit of unrealistic beauty standards and the stigma attached to weight can exacerbate stress and trauma, especially in those vulnerable to BED. A culture that prizes thinness and shames those who don't conform creates an environment ripe for disordered eating.

The narrative of trauma and stress as it relates to BED is woven with the threads of resilience and hope. While the scars of trauma and the weight of stress may never fully disappear, their role in binge eating can be addressed, providing a path towards recovery and empowerment. With this knowledge, individuals can begin to dismantle the hold that stress and trauma have on their eating behaviors, rebuilding their relationship with food upon a foundation of self-awareness and self-compassion.

As we close this section, it's important to remember: healing is not linear, nor is it a race. It's an individual journey that varies from one person to another. Recognition of the role stress and trauma play in BED is a crucial step towards understanding and treating this complex disorder. With the right support and treatment strategies, those affected can regain control and lead more balanced, fulfilling lives.

Chapter 5:
The Physiology of Binge Eating

As we delve deeper into the labyrinth of Binge Eating Disorder (BED), our journey brings us to the critical understanding of the physiological underpinnings that fuel this complex condition. At the core of BED lies a tangled web of hunger hormones and brain chemistry that can sabotage the most earnest attempts at self-control. Yet, it's not just about hunger; dopamine, the neurotransmitter associated with pleasure, often becomes a key player in the cycle of binge eating, reinforcing the compulsive behavior despite negative consequences. This potent biological cocktail can leave individuals feeling powerless in the face of their own biology. To combat these physiological forces, one must first acknowledge the profound impact physical health has on the disorder, recognizing that fluctuations in blood sugar levels and nutritional imbalances can exacerbate cravings and binges. In understanding this cycle, those who struggle with BED can find powerful insights and leverage in their journey towards recovery, harnessing knowledge to break free from the physiological chains that bind them to this relentless eating pattern.

Hunger Hormones and Brain Chemistry

In unraveling the complexity of Binge Eating Disorder (BED), it becomes crucial to delve into a largely invisible but powerful arena: the interplay of hunger hormones and brain chemistry. As science peers into the biological underpinnings of this disorder, the roles of hormones such as ghrelin and leptin, along with the neurotransmitters that govern mood and appetite, come into sharp focus.

Ghrelin, often dubbed the 'hunger hormone,' elevates before meals and drops after eating, signaling the brain to initiate food intake. It's a call to action, an alert that the body needs sustenance. In persons with BED, this signaling can become skewed, creating a false sensation of hunger or an overwhelmingly powerful urge to eat, contributing to the cycle of binging. Conversely, leptin—the 'satiety hormone'—produced by adipose tissue, tells the brain when it's time to put down the fork. Disrupted leptin signals could mean that individuals don't feel satisfied and may continue to eat past the point of fullness.

Dopamine, the 'reward' neurotransmitter, also plays a pivotal role in BED. This chemical messenger is released when we experience pleasure, which includes the act of eating, particularly foods high in fat or sugar. A hearty dish or a slice of cake can light up the brain's pleasure centers akin to other rewarding activities. However, in BED, the dopamine system may be overly receptive or overly released in response to food, making the experience of eating more rewarding, and thus more compulsive than for others.

Another neurotransmitter, serotonin, is often associated with feelings of wellbeing and happiness. Low levels of serotonin are linked with mood disorders and, notably, may cause an increased appetite for carbohydrates. This craving can perpetuate the cycle of binging, particularly on sweet or starchy foods that spike serotonin levels temporarily, only to crash later, making it a significant player in the BED puzzle.

Why does this matter? Understanding the hormonal and chemical fluctuations that drive hunger and mood is crucial in addressing BED at its roots. As scientists continue to study the hormonal and brain chemistry abnormalities in those with BED, we embark on a promising journey that might soon provide more targeted treatments and interventions. Imagine a future where medical advancements could recalibrate these signals to reduce the overpowering urges to binge.

For instance, medications that alter the function of these hormones or neurotransmitters are becoming potential game-changers in managing BED. While not without complexities, these pharmacological therapies signal a new horizon for treatment—one that directly intervenes in the bio-chemical cascade leading to bouts of uncontrolled eating. Tailoring treatments to address the hormonal imbalances and neurotransmitter activities unique to each individual could transform the landscape of BED therapy.

Addressing hunger hormone imbalances can also be approached through lifestyle modifications. As the field burgeons, nutrition and exercise have been shown to impact the production and effectiveness of these hormones. Mindful eating practices and balanced diets can help stabilize ghrelin and leptin levels, while regular physical activity can optimize the reward feedback loop regulated by dopamine.

Embedding knowledge of hormones and brain chemistry into therapeutic strategies, such as Cognitive-Behavioral Therapy (CBT) and Interpersonal Psychotherapy (IPT), can enhance the effectiveness of these treatments. A more profound awareness of how and why cravings occur can empower individuals to intercept the urge to binge before it gains unstoppable momentum. Psypiatrists and therapists can guide patients through cognitive strategies that strengthen the mind's resilience against the misfiring of hunger and reward pathways.

The complexity of BED is compounded by the fact that hormones and neurotransmitters do not act in isolation. Other factors, such as genetics, stress, previous trauma, and one's emotional state, intermingle with these biological mechanisms. For instance, chronic stress can exacerbate ghrelin and cortisol levels, pushing individuals toward comfort eating. This demonstrates the necessity of a holistic approach in treatment—where both mind and body are addressed concurrently.

Despite our growing knowledge, it's crucial to recognize the need for individualized approaches. Each person's chemical makeup is unique, and so too is their experience with BED. What can trigger an overwhelming desire to binge in one person might not have the same effect on another. Hence, personalization is the cornerstone of successful treatment, integrating scientific understanding with empathy and psychological insight.

We know that BED manifests not only in the psyche but also in the body's fundamental biology. To restore balance, we must employ a synergy of approaches that cater to both aspects. Multidisciplinary teams—including dictitians, psychologists, endocrinologists, and psychiatrists—need to work together to craft and implement comprehensive management plans.

In navigating through the journey of understanding and ultimately conquering BED, patients and professionals alike must acknowledge the importance of patience and perseverance. Changes in brain chemistry and hormonal balance will not occur overnight, and strategies must have room for adjustment as insights develop and as individuals respond to treatment.

We stand on the brink of understanding the biological underpinnings of appetite, hunger, and compulsion in unprecedented ways. This knowledge beckons us forward, promising new and improved treatments for those grappling with BED. It's a call steeped in scientific rationale and imbued with hope—a combination that can spur individuals on towards recovery and a healthier future.

In closing, it is essential to reiterate that while hormones and brain chemistry play a significant role in BED, they are but one part of it. A compassionate and comprehensive approach to therapy, underscored by cutting-edge research and its application, can offer the most effective support to those facing the challenges of BED.

The Impact on Physical Health

The journey through understanding the intricacies of Binge Eating Disorder (BED) brings us to a critical aspect that warrants thorough exploration: the impact on physical health. Often overshadowed by the psychological facets of the disorder, the physiological repercussions of BED present a myriad of complexities that undeniably transform the body.

First and foremost, it is essential to acknowledge the significant strain that binge eating episodes place on the digestive system. The abdomen is not designed to accommodate the large quantities of food typically consumed during a binge. This can lead to uncomfortable distention, acid reflux, and in more severe cases, gastric rupture - a life-threatening condition. The episodic stress placed on these organs cannot be understated, and chronic complications such as gastroesophageal reflux disease (GERD) remain a serious concern for individuals with BED.

Additionally, BED is intrinsically linked with weight fluctuations and often obesity. The rapid intake of high-calorie foods during binges can result in metabolic disturbances, causing the body to store fat more readily. This increased weight can place undue stress on the cardiovascular system, heightening the risk for high blood pressure, heart disease, and stroke. The risk could be decreased through an integrative approach focused on addressing both the eating behavior and its physiological effects.

Moving beyond the cardiovascular system, the endocrine system also bears the brunt of BED's impact. The disorder can severely disrupt insulin regulation, with episodes of overeating exacerbating the body's ability to manage blood sugar levels effectively. This imbalance may pave the way for Type 2 diabetes, a common comorbidity linked with BED that not only demands meticulous lifelong management but also increases the risk of additional health complications.

Equally, the skeletal system feels the reverberations of BED's physical toll. Excessive body weight can lead to joint pain, deterioration, and the possible onset of osteoarthritis. The ability of the body's frame to support itself is compromised, leading to a reduction in mobility and a decreased quality of life.

Perhaps less frequently discussed are the repercussions that BED can have on the body's largest organ: the skin. Poor nutrition and the stress associated with BED can result in skin issues such as acne, eczema, or other dermatological conditions. The skin often reflects the internal state of the body, and its maladies warrant equal concern and attention.

Moreover, the risk for certain types of cancer increases with the presence of obesity and unhealthy eating patterns characteristic of BED. The interplay between diet, weight, and cancer risk solidifies the need for a greater understanding and intervention aimed at mitigating these dangers.

BED is also linked with potential reproductive health issues. In women, the disorder can contribute to irregular menstrual cycles and complications with fertility (Kessler et al., 2016). These impacts can have profound implications for those wishing to conceive, further emphasizing the extensive scope of BED's reach on health.

And let us not overlook the respiratory system. Obesity associated with BED can lead to sleep apnea, a condition where breathing repeatedly stops and starts during sleep. Sleep apnea not only hinders the body's restorative processes but also its daily functionality, leading to fatigue and further impacting the body's overall health.

Equally disconcerting is the potential for liver damage. Non-alcoholic fatty liver disease can result from the accumulation of fat in liver cells—a noteworthy risk for those with BED. This condition can progress to liver inflammation, fibrosis, and cirrhosis if unaddressed.

A crucial aspect of physical health that is negatively influenced by BED is immune function. The relationship between diet and immunity is complex and intimate. A consistently poor diet, replete with the overconsumption of processed and sugary foods, can impair the body's immune response, rendering an individual with BED more susceptible to infections and illnesses.

We must also contemplate the impact of BED on oral health. The high incidence of sugary and acidic food consumption can result in dental caries, enamel erosion, and in serious cases, tooth loss. The condition demands an integrated health approach, considering not only the individual's eating habits but their entire well-being.

Fulfilling the tenet that knowledge is power, understanding these health implications inform us of the critical need for comprehensive treatment strategies. Targeted interventions can mitigate the multitude of risks posed by BED's physical health impacts. Truly, recovery involves not only overcoming psychological hurdles but also embracing holistic practices that fortify physical health.

In conclusion, the impact of Binge Eating Disorder on physical health extends far beyond a singular aspect of the human body. It has the capacity to infiltrate every system, leaving a wake of potential health concerns that must be considered with earnest attention. The dissemination of this knowledge positions us to more effectively combat BED—and in doing so, foster a future where the physical repercussions are no longer a daunting inevitability but a challenge that can be met with unwavering resolve and informed strategy.

The Cycle of Binge Eating

The cycle of binge eating is an entrapping sequence, a pattern of behavior typified by an overwhelming urge to consume large amounts of food followed by feelings of shame and a promise to abstain, which eventually leads back to bingeing. It's a slippery slope and understanding this process is crucial for those who are trapped in its relentless rotation.

Diving into the core, binge eating episodes often begin with an irresistible impulse. Research suggests this initial surge might result from a combination of hormonal imbalances and psychological factors.

This biological vulnerability is then exacerbated by psychological distress. Emotional triggers such as stress, anxiety, or depression often act as catalysts. It's a cycle that's as physiological as it is psychological, underscoring the complexity of BED.

Once the binge begins, there's often a disconnection from one's sense of fullness and satiety. Eaters may eat rapidly and to the point of discomfort, experiencing a loss of control and inability to stop eating. This phase can feel hypnotic, an auto-pilot mode where awareness of quantity and satiation is absent. It is testament to the power of disrupted brain circuitry among binge eaters, which impedes their ability to regulate food intake.

Subsuming the immediate gratification from eating is the ensuing wave of guilt. A binger may be flooded with self-criticism and a harsh internal dialogue. The regret prompts resolutions to make a change, vows that often include strict diets or compensatory behaviors like excessive exercise. But these promises can be unrealistic and unsustainable, inadvertently sowing the seeds for another cycle.

Restriction follows, often framed as the solution to the 'problem' of binge eating. The imposition of severe dietary rules in an attempt to control weight or to compensate for overeating can trigger a starvation response in the body, intensifying the physiological drive to binge eat.

After a period of restriction, an individual often experiences a lowered psychological resilience, as decrements in mood and increased preoccupation with food set in. Emotions run high, stress escalates, and the urge to find solace in food becomes irresistible once again, leading to a repeat of the binge episode.

The emotional aftermath of a binge can shift one's self-image. With each perceived 'failure', the individual's confidence in their ability to change decreases, exacerbating feelings of helplessness and perpetuating the negative self-image that often accompanies BED.

Throughout the binge eating cycle, there are also social impacts. Isolation becomes common as individuals may avoid social situations for fear of episodes occurring or judgment, further hindering recovery by reducing the potential for social support.

In order to break this punishing cycle, a multifaceted approach is essential. Recognizing the pattern is just the first step. Subsequent measures require confronting the underlying emotional triggers, modifying dysfunctional eating patterns, and, importantly, instilling a compassionate self-view that tolerates imperfections.

Medications such as SSRIs have shown some efficacy in reducing binge eating behaviors by addressing underlying mood disturbances. However, medications should be considered as part of a comprehensive treatment plan rather than a standalone remedy.

Therapeutic interventions like Cognitive-Behavioral Therapy (CBT) have proven effective in disrupting the binge eating cycle by helping individuals develop coping mechanisms that don't involve food. CBT focuses on challenging and changing unhelpful cognitive distortions and behaviors, and improving emotional regulation.

Along with CBT, other therapies like Interpersonal Psychotherapy (IPT) and Dialectical Behavior Therapy (DBT) address the relational and self-regulation aspects respectively, providing strategies to manage the emotions and relationships that often factor into the cycle of binge eating.

Lastly, a sustainable, nurturing approach towards dieting, one that promotes balance rather than restriction, can help stabilize eating patterns. This may involve working with dietitians to establish a healthy relationship with food, as opposed to adopting extreme dietary measures.

Understanding the cycle of binge eating isn't just about dissecting its phases; it's about recognizing that each element is interwoven with physiological, psychological, and social fibers. By addressing the cycle holistically, individuals with BED can embark on a journey towards recovery, which, though challenging, leads to a life beyond the devastating loops of binge eating.

Chapter 6:
Prevention of BED

As we transition from understanding the physiological underpinnings of binge eating disorder (BED) discussed in Chapter 5, we are now poised to forge a crucial armor against its insidious onset: prevention. Illuminating the shadows of ignorance through awareness and education is a pivotal step, akin to wielding a torch that scatters the specters of misconception and shame. Crafting a bulwark of support is not a lonesome venture; it requires the collective strength of families, friends, and healthcare providers, reflecting the ethos that the whole is indeed greater than the sum of its parts. Instilling a preventative mindset reverberates with principle, for it is not merely about evading the disorder but nurturing a life that throbs with vigor and resilience. In the melange of armor and mindset, one discovers tools both potent and profound—strategies encapsulated by research that unfalteringly animate our path to stifle BED before its seed takes root. While subsequent chapters will dissect further intricacies of managing and treating BED, it is here, in the realm of prevention, where we chart the course away from potential struggles and toward a horizon of well-being.

Awareness and Education

Embarking on the journey of overcoming Binge Eating Disorder (BED), one cannot overstate the value of awareness and education. Prior chapters have dissected the nature of BED, it's diagnosis, and the intimately woven psychological and physiological traits that contribute to this complex condition. It's now critical to center on how increased knowledge and consciousness can serve as cornerstones in the proactive attempt to prevent BED's onset and progression. Firstly, education empowers individuals with the understanding that BED is a legitimate health condition that warrants attention and care.

Stigma, sadly, often remains entrenched in discussions about eating disorders, causing many to suffer in silence. By improving the quality and accessibility of information, we can dismantle misconceptions surrounding BED, helping those affected feel seen and supported rather than shamed. Furthermore, awareness campaigns, educational programs, and resource dissemination to schools, workplaces, and health institutions can facilitate early detection and encourage individuals to seek help promptly.

Education can also amplify the importance of nuanced conversations around food, body image, and health. As we uncover the shared narratives that underscore the struggle against BED, it becomes essential to challenge damaging societal norms and narratives that often contribute to the disorder's development. Educational endeavors seek to create environments where diverse body types are respected and where the relationship with food is centered on nourishment and well-being, rather than restriction and fear.

Undoubtedly, equipping healthcare professionals with comprehensive training on BED can enhance the quality of support offered to those in need. Clinicians familiar with the telltale signs and contributing factors of BED are better positioned to engage in empathetic dialogue with individuals exhibiting early signs of the disorder. This specialized knowledge is pivotal in fostering a therapeutic alliance that prioritizes the person's holistic health, above and beyond weight management or clinical symptomatology alone.

Finally, education is a springboard for advocacy. Knowledge enables those impacted by BED, and their allies, to champion for policy changes and societal shifts that value mental health parity and the de-stigmatization of all eating disorders. As awareness seeds change, it becomes an unstoppable force, empowering individuals to transform personal struggles into collective triumphs against BED.

Building a Support System

In navigating the challenges of Binge Eating Disorder (BED), forging a resilient support system is both a beacon of hope and a practical necessity. Studies have shown that social support plays a pivotal role in the treatment and recovery from various eating disorders, including BED. Yet, recognizing you need others and actively seeking their support requires courage and a willingness to let go of the insidious pride that often accompanies the solitary battle against eating disorders.

Creating this support system starts with identifying individuals in your life who are understanding, non-judgmental, and genuinely concerned about your wellbeing. This may include family members, friends, or even coworkers. Additionally, healthcare providers, therapists, and dietitians are a crucial component of the support network, offering not only counseling and medical advice but also a structured treatment plan. However, the quality of these relationships trumps quantity; a few close, trusted supporters will be more effective than a larger, less intimate group.

Participation in support groups, both in-person and online, offers a collective sense of understanding and shared experiences. These groups can alleviate the feeling of isolation that many with BED experience. The power of shared narratives and learned wisdom from those who have walked a similar path can inspire and offer tangible strategies for managing the disorder. Furthermore, mutual support groups foster a sense of accountability which is invaluable during the recovery journey.

While building a personal support system, it's also essential to develop self-support strategies. These strategies aim to fortify your inner resilience and enable you to provide self-compassion and understanding. Self-care routines, mindfulness practice, and pursuits that foster a positive self-image all contribute to this self-reliant aspect of your support system. This dimension of support empowers an individual with BED to handle stressors constructively without defaulting to binge eating as a coping mechanism.

In conclusion, constructing a robust support system is a significant step toward preventing and managing Binge Eating Disorder. It's a dynamic interplay of external and internal resources tailored to meet the unique needs of the individual. Embracing support from others, cultivating self-support, and engaging with professional care creates an ecosystem of recovery, essential for long-term success. Building this system may not be easy, but its impact on your journey to recovery is immeasurable, offering not just a lifeline, but also a path forward through the often-turbulent waters of BED.

Creating a Preventative Mindset

As we move through our exploration of Binge Eating Disorder (BED), it becomes increasingly clear that cultivation of a preventative mindset is crucial. Although BED can feel overwhelming, adopting a proactive stance empowers individuals to navigate the complexities of the disorder with strength and resilience. A preventative mindset embodies the anticipation of potential triggers, the establishment of supportive habits, and the balance between vigilance and adaptability.

Firstly, understanding one's personal triggers is fundamental to prevention. These can range from emotional states to specific social scenarios, and recognizing them allows for the implementation of strategies to mitigate their impact. It's also essential to align these strategies with evidence-based practices. For instance, regular mindfulness exercises have been shown to reduce the frequency and severity of binge eating episodes by fostering an awareness of bodily cues and emotional states. By making these practices a routine, one cultivates a mindfulness that serves as a barricade against the onset of a binge.

Another key aspect of forming a preventative mindset is to integrate education with actionable habits. Knowledge is a form of power that allows individuals to distinguish between unhealthy eating patterns and nourishing practices. Through education, individuals can grasp the physiological underpinnings of hunger and satiety, enabling them to align their eating habits with their body's natural cues. Furthermore, this knowledge empowers individuals to make informed decisions about their nutrition and lifestyle, which can reinforce their preventative strategies.

Building a support system is an indispensable component of prevention. A preventative mindset isn't an isolated perspective but thrives in an environment backed by understanding peers, healthcare professionals, and possibly even a mentor who has navigated BED's turbulent waters. A connection with others who provide compassion and insight strengthens one's resolve and furnishes a sense of shared experience, thereby mitigating feelings of isolation that can precipitate binge eating behaviors.

Lastly, adaptability is a defining characteristic of a preventative mindset. As experiences and circumstances evolve, so must one's approach to prevention. What works today may not be as effective tomorrow, and the readiness to adapt one's methods is key to long-term success in managing BED. The interplay of knowledge, self-awareness, and support culminates in an adaptable and robust preventative mindset, carving a pathway through the complexities of BED and toward a brighter, more controlled relationship with food and self.

Chapter 7:
The Emotional Landscape of BED

In the previous chapters, we have navigated through the clinical and physiological terrains of Binge Eating Disorder (BED). Now, we delve into the multifaceted emotional landscape that underpins BED's daunting presence. Beneath the surface of this disorder lies a labyrinth of emotions—pain, shame, and guilt interlace with the threads of coping mechanisms, forming a complex range of psychological challenges. It's essential to discern the nuanced ways in which individuals with BED relate to their emotions and how these internal experiences can precipitate a binge episode. As we explore the terrain of emotional turmoil, we recognize that food often becomes an anesthetic, temporarily dulling the acute sensitivity to life's distresses. However, within this chapter, we not only map out the craggy contours of emotional upheaval but also illuminate pathways to emotional resilience. We examine strategies such as mindfulness and emotional regulation—promising tools empowering people to traverse their emotions without succumbing to the compulsion of binge eating. Addressing the intertwined co-occurring disorders is also paramount, as they can exacerbate BED symptoms and hinder recovery. Mastering the emotional landscape of BED isn't a conquest but a journey of compassionate self-discovery, guiding one towards a holistic reconciliation with food and feelings.

Coping with Feelings Without Food

Embracing the challenge to manage emotions without the crutch of food requires a purposeful shift in perspective. The concept of emotional eating, using food to soothe or suppress feelings, is a recognized hallmark in those struggling with Binge Eating Disorder (BED). Herein lies the crux of transcending the disorder, where the journey toward healing takes a pivotal turn. You've recognized the emotional triggers and identified them as precursors to your binges. Now, let's delve into the constructive ways to process these emotions without turning to food as a source of temporary relief.

Firstly, the art of mindfulness has proven to be a cornerstone in altering one's response to emotional upheaval. Engaging in mindfulness means to be wholly present in the moment without judgment, to recognize an oncoming wave of emotion, acknowledge it, but let it pass without having to feed it, literally. Techniques such as focused breathing or guided imagery can act as anchors, preventing you from being swept away by feelings of sadness, stress, or boredom. The emphasis here is on 'focused' – by narrowing your awareness to your breath or a mental image, you create a buffer between your emotions and your immediate reactions.

Another technique to employ is cognitive restructuring, a skill that can be honed with or without the aid of a therapist. By challenging the thoughts that typically lead to a binge, such as feelings of inadequacy or abandonment, and replacing them with truths and affirmations, you can begin to disentangle yourself from the compulsion to eat in response to emotion. Positive self-talk can be incredibly powerful. Instead of saying "I'm overwhelmed, I need to eat," you could say, "I'm overwhelmed, but I am capable of handling this." This seemingly small linguistic shift can signal a massive change in coping strategy.

Journaling serves as an emotional release valve, providing a safe vessel for your thoughts and feelings. The act of writing can transform amorphous worries and nebulous sadness into tangible challenges that can be faced and managed. It's a way to confront your feelings head-on rather than masking them with food, and over time, it can strengthen your emotional resilience. A consistent journaling habit can make all the difference, as it becomes a daily ritual for self-reflection and self-soothing (Enhanced and Crippled by Technology, 2022).

Lastly, developing a robust support system is invaluable when navigating the tumultuous seas of emotion. Surrounding yourself with people who understand, empathize, and encourage your journey can make an ocean of difference. Peer support groups, therapy sessions, and even online communities can offer you a sense of companionship and shared struggle, ensuring you know you're not facing these challenges in isolation. The collective wisdom and strength of a support network can propel you toward newfound strategies for emotional regulation and provide you with a diverse toolkit to resist the pull of emotional eating.

Mindfulness and Emotional Regulation

is a crucial component in the journey of understanding and combating Binge Eating Disorder (BED). While previous sections have laid the groundwork by identifying and diagnosing BED, this current exploration allows individuals to dive deeper into effective ways of managing emotion-driven eating behaviors.

Mindfulness, as the term suggests, involves being fully present and engaged in the moment without harsh judgment. When applied to eating, mindfulness encourages an awareness of the physical and emotional sensations associated with food consumption. It counters the automatic, stressful thought patterns that often lead to binge eating episodes. For individuals with BED, adopting a mindful approach can help to identify emotional triggers and create a buffer between feelings and actions, allowing space for more thoughtful responses to emotional distress.

However, the connection between mindfulness and emotional regulation expands beyond mere awareness. Emotional regulation is a person's ability to effectively manage and respond to an emotional experience. It's fundamental in halting the cycle where intense emotions trigger binge eating as a coping mechanism. By recognizing and accepting their emotions without immediately resorting to food, individuals can cultivate resilience and healthier coping strategies.

Integrating mindfulness practices such as meditation, deep breathing, or yoga helps individuals develop a stronger connection between mind and body. This connection fosters a heightened awareness that can defuse the intensity of negative emotions linked to binge eating. Clinical studies have indicated that mindfulness techniques can significantly improve self-regulation.

Moreover, the role of emotional regulation strategies in mindfulness cannot be overstated. Techniques such as reappraisal and cognitive defusion help change the way an individual reacts to their thoughts and feelings. Instead of immediately seeking comfort in food, they can step back, examine the validity of their emotions, and choose a healthier response.

Another aspect of emotion regulation pertains to the development of distress tolerance skills. It's not uncommon for individuals with BED to perceive certain emotional states as intolerable and to use binge eating as an escape. By building distress tolerance, they learn to sit with discomfort without the need for immediate resolution, which is often where binge eating fits into the picture.

Training in mindfulness and emotional regulation can take time, and it demands patience and consistent practice. Individuals may find it helpful to attend guided sessions or use digital tools designed to foster mindfulness, gradually incorporating these into their daily routine and, specifically, their approach towards food and eating.

As individuals become more skilled in mindfulness and emotional regulation, they might notice a diminishing need to engage in binge eating. The space that these strategies create allows for more intentional and nourishing choices, both nutritionally and emotionally. Mindfulness fosters a compassionate self-awareness that empowers individuals to address their needs constructively, thereby easing the compulsion to find solace in overeating.

Addressing Co-occurring Disorders

has become an essential component in the treatment of Binge Eating Disorder (BED). It's imperative to understand that BED rarely exists in isolation. Research has frequently illuminated the comorbidity between BED and a range of psychological disorders, from depression and anxiety to substance abuse and personality disorders. Addressing these co-occurring disorders is not just a matter of comprehensive care; it's a necessity for achieving sustained recovery and improving the quality of life for those affected by BED.

First and foremost, it's important for individuals and healthcare providers to recognize the high rate of dual diagnoses in individuals with BED. This recognition necessitates a treatment plan that is multi-faceted and integrative, focusing not solely on the symptoms of BED but also on the underlying co-occurring disorders. Treating BED in tandem with other mental health disorders requires a patient-centered approach, often involving a team of specialists including therapists, psychiatrists, dietitians, and primary care physicians. An integrated treatment plan may include cognitive-behavioral therapy, known for its effectiveness in treating a variety of psychological disorders, as well as targeted medications to manage specific symptoms.

Substance abuse, an example of a co-occurring disorder with BED, can present unique challenges. The use of substances may serve as a maladaptive coping mechanism for managing the distress associated with binge eating. It's crucial that interventions for substance abuse are incorporated into the treatment plan. Behavioral therapies, such as motivational interviewing and contingency management, alongside support groups, can provide individuals coping with both BED and substance abuse the tools they need to break free from the cycle of addiction and develop healthier coping strategies.

Anxiety and depression frequently accompany BED, and they can exacerbate the struggle with eating behaviors. Addressing these emotional disorders is essential to reduce the likelihood of binge episodes and create a more stable emotional environment. A combination of psychotherapy, such as interpersonal therapy or dialectical behavior therapy, and pharmacotherapy, including selective serotonin reuptake inhibitors (SSRIs), can be effective in treating co-occurring anxiety and depression alongside BED. Such treatments aim to equip individuals with the skills to regulate emotions, improve interpersonal relationships, and mitigate the depressive symptoms that can be potent triggers for binge eating.

Chapter 8:
Proactive Strategies for Managing BED

Navigating the complexities of Binge Eating Disorder (BED) necessitates not just understanding and acceptance but actionable tactics that arm individuals with the means to assert control over their eating behaviors. As we delve into Chapter 8, we recognize that proactive strategies form the cornerstone of managing BED effectively. Nutritional guidance, structured not as an austere regimen but as a sustainable meal plan, equips one with the blueprint to circumvent the chaos of binge episodes. A judicious blend of satiety and satisfaction can redraw the relationship with food from adversarial to amicable. Though developing healthy eating habits is often laden with challenges, incremental adjustments over time can encode a new normal, emphasizing balance over deprivation (Jones & Williams, 2021). Additionally, the role of physical activity transcends mere caloric balance; it is the vestiges of empowerment, the restored communion of body and mind, fostering resilience against the urge to binge. The strategies outlined in this chapter coalesce into a formidable defense, not merely to cope with BED, but to thrive in spite of it.

Nutritional Guidance and Meal Planning

Embarking on the journey of overcoming Binge Eating Disorder (BED) requires a holistic and evidence-based approach, and central to this quest is the role of tailored nutrition and thoughtful meal planning. Evidently, the simple notion of eating 'healthily' becomes complex amidst the throes of BED, where the relationship with food is tumultuous.

Nutrition for individuals with BED isn't merely about choosing the right foods; it's about establishing a framework that supports consistent, mindful eating habits. Guiding principles should include balanced macronutrient intake and an understanding of how certain foods can trigger binge eating episodes. A practical place to start is with the planning of regular, nutritionally dense meals and snacks to stave off impulsivity and the physiological cues that spark binges.

Meal planning is a strategic pillar in this rehabilitation. A weekly meal plan serves as a map; it comforts the mind with a predictable structure while ensuring that decision fatigue—so often a foe in the face of food—doesn't become an incitement to binge. By pre-determining what and when to eat, the individual with BED can focus on cultivating a more harmonious relationship with food, one that affirms autonomy rather than chaos.

The composition of meals should lean towards foods with a low glycemic index, providing a stable release of energy that curbs the hunger peaks and troughs associated with craving cycles. Additionally, incorporating adequate fiber, healthy fats, and protein can contribute to satiety and reduce the likelihood of overeating (Mazurek & Yetman, 2020). However, it's essential that this guidance doesn't morph into rigid dietary control as that can inadvertently fuel the cycle of restriction and bingeing.

It is important to remember that no single meal plan is one-size-fits-all. Personal tastes, allergies, physical activity levels, and nutritional needs will inform the customizable nature of meal plans. This flexibility is empowering; it garners a sense of control that so often feels lost in individuals struggling with BED. Nutritional therapy can thus be an integral part of recovery, constructing a healthy and sustainable eating pattern that normalizes portion sizes and respects the body's natural cues.

Equally vital to successful meal planning is the inclusion of pleasure and variation. Dietary monotony can be a subtle trap, leading back to the very behaviors meal planning sought to avert. By introducing a diverse array of flavors and cuisines, the pleasure of eating can be rekindled within safe and nourishing parameters. Exploring new recipes and cooking techniques not only engenders an enriching relationship with food but also dilutes the fixation on consuming 'forbidden' items that often precipitate a binge.

When creating a meal plan, individuals are encouraged to engage in intentional eating, which involves being present and mindful during meals. Slowing down, chewing thoroughly, and removing distractions can enhance the body's ability to signal fullness and satisfaction effectively. In doing so, mealtime becomes a refuge of deliberate nourishment rather than a battleground of compulsion.

It is crucial to acknowledge setbacks as they come and treat them as opportunities for learning rather than failures. Stressful days or unexpected events might lead to deviations from the meal plan. The key is not perfection but resilience and the resolve to return to structured eating without self-reprimand. The focus must remain on long-term patterns and progress, rather than isolated occurrences.

As nutrition takes its rightful place in BED recovery, the individual is empowered to redefine their relationship with food. It is not the enemy, nor is it a source of instant gratification, but rather a sustainer of life and health. Armed with a thoughtful, flexible meal plan, individuals with BED can step boldly in the direction of safe, satisfying, and self-affirming eating behaviors.

In summary, the essence of nutritional guidance and meal planning as a cornerstone in the recovery from BED is to foster a sustainable, positive relationship with food and eating. A supportive, scientifically sound, and compassionate approach to meal planning can make an appreciable difference in both short-term management and long-term recovery from binge eating behaviors.

Developing Healthy Eating Habits

as part of managing Binge Eating Disorder (BED) is crucial for both recovery and sustaining long-term health. It's about creating a balance of nourishment where food becomes an ally rather than an adversary.

Firstly, establishing structured meal times can create a framework that reduces the uncertainty around eating, a common trigger for binges. A regular pattern of eating throughout the day helps to regulate hunger hormones like ghrelin and leptin, which signal hunger and fullness, respectively. These hormones can often be disrupted in individuals with BED, leading to challenges in recognizing true hunger cues. Consistency in meal timing aids in normalizing these signals and reduces the likelihood of mistaking emotional hunger for physical hunger.

It's also important to integrate a variety of foods into the diet to ensure that all macronutrient and micronutrient needs are met. The goal is to consume a balanced mix of carbohydrates, proteins, and fats, along with an abundance of fruits, vegetables, and whole grains. This approach promotes satiety and helps in stabilizing blood sugar levels— an essential factor since fluctuations can contribute to cravings and binge eating.

Moreover, developing a mindful eating practice can enhance the awareness of the body's hunger and fullness signals, as well as the sensory experience of eating. By being present during meals, individuals can slow down the eating process, leading to better digestion and more enjoyment of their food. Being mindful also means acknowledging and respecting the body's satiety signals, which can help prevent overeating. It calls for a moment of pause, to check in with one's feelings, and to identify if the desire to eat stems from physical hunger or emotional need.

Fostering a non-judgmental attitude towards food is also vital. Labeling certain foods as "off-limits" can create a sense of deprivation that fuels the binge cycle. It's healthier to view all foods as permissible within the framework of an overall balanced diet—an approach advocated by the concept of intuitive eating. This promotes a healthier relationship with food, characterized by choosing foods for nourishment and satisfaction rather than out of restriction or fear.

The Importance of Physical Activity

In examining the multifaceted approach to managing Binge Eating Disorder (BED), one cannot overlook the critical role of physical activity as a proactive strategy. While the earlier sections have laid down the conceptual framework of BED, it's equally important to understand how integrating a consistent exercise regimen can be transformative for those struggling with this disorder.

Research consistently underscores the benefits of exercise, not just for physical fitness, but also for mental well-being. This is particularly relevant for those with BED, where the intertwining of physical and emotional health can create a complex web of challenges. Engaging in regular physical activity can catalyze a myriad of positive effects—reducing stress, enhancing mood, and improving self-esteem—each of which can be a powerful counter to the impulses of binge eating.

Under the gripping cycles of BED, the body often endures intense fluctuations in energy intake. Exercise may help to stabilize these variances by improving metabolic function and insulin sensitivity. This increased efficiency can lead to a more balanced and regulated energy state, weakening one of the physiological drivers of binge behavior.

Contrary to the notion of exercise as a punitive measure for calorie-burning, we must adopt a different perspective: physical activity as empowerment. Selecting activities that one enjoys can transform exercise from an obligation to a rewarding experience. This mindset encourages a sustainable, affirmative relationship with one's body. The underlying aim is not solely weight management, but rather, fostering a deeper connection with and appreciation for one's own physical capabilities and resilience.

Furthermore, physical activity serves as an anchor for structure in a person's daily life. This structure establishes a rhythm and gives a sense of control and predictability. Having a regular schedule for exercise can provide a constructive focus and a break from the obsessive food thoughts that frequently accompany BED. Moving one's focus from food to fitness, even if just for a portion of the day, can deliver a crucial reprieve for someone entrenched in a cycle of binge eating.

It is also pertinent to recognize the social dimensions that physical activities often embrace. Whether it's team sports, group fitness classes, or walk-and-talks with friends, these shared experiences can reinforce a sense of community and belonging. For individuals coping with BED, these connections are invaluable. They afford avenues for social support, which has been shown to significantly affect recovery outcomes.

Yet, it's essential to approach physical activity with caution for those with BED. The exercise regimen should be balanced and moderate, to avoid the potential pitfall of obsessive exercise, which could simply replace one compulsive behavior with another. A thoughtful, measured approach that consults healthcare professionals can ensure that activity levels are conducive to healing rather than harm.

In essence, physical activity is not merely a complement but a cornerstone in the holistic treatment of BED. Its benefits permeate beyond the corporeal, enriching the mind, mending the emotions, and strengthening the spirit. This trinity of wellness—physical, mental, emotional—is the crucible within which recovery is forged, and through which a life of balance can be attained and sustained.

Encouraging those with BED to incorporate physical activity into their lives is not a simple directive; it requires understanding the nuanced layers of the disorder, compassion for the struggles involved, and a commitment to gentle encouragement over time. The aim should always be to guide, not push; to inspire, not compel. This approach ensures that physical activity is a choice made with self-love—as essential to well-being as therapy and nutritional guidance—and not just another expectation to live up to.

At the crossroads of an individual's journey with BED, where despair can overshadow hope, it's the act of moving—one step, one breath, one heartbeat at a time—that can help reclaim one's power over the disorder. Exercise is more than mere movement; it's a language of self-care that speaks of strength and resilience. It tells the story of a body not defined by binge eating, but redefined in every stride, lift, and stretch towards recovery.

Chapter 9:
Treatments of BED

In the pursuit of reclaiming control from Binge Eating Disorder (BED), the beacon of hope shines predominantly on evidence-based treatments, capable of navigating individuals through the tempest of this condition. Cognitive-Behavioral Therapy (CBT), the gold standard in psychological treatments, offers a structured approach that dissects the relationship between thoughts, behaviors, and feelings, with proven efficacy in mitigating binge-eating episodes. Alongside CBT, Interpersonal Psychotherapy (IPT) warrants a significant place by addressing personal relationships and the underlying social factors contributing to BED, highlighting the profound influence of interpersonal disputes and role transitions on eating behaviors. Moreover, embracing a scientific avenue, medication, and pharmacotherapy have also demonstrated their capacity to alleviate BED symptoms, with some medications receiving FDA approval specifically for this disorder, showing a reduction in the frequency of binge eating and an improvement in associated psychiatric conditions. Constantly evolving, these treatments quintessentially represent the nexus of hope and recovery.

Cognitive-Behavioral Therapy (CBT)

Continuing our journey toward understanding and treating Binge Eating Disorder (BED), let us delve into one of its most effective forms of psychological intervention: Cognitive-Behavioral Therapy (CBT). This evidence-based approach is at the forefront of treatment strategies for BED, providing structured and skill-based therapy that targets the dysfunctional eating behaviors and thought patterns which typify this condition. Fundamentally, CBT operates on the premise that psychological problems are in part due to maladaptive thinking and learned patterns of unhelpful behavior. In BED, CBT seeks to dismantle these patterns by teaching individuals more adaptive ways of thinking and behaving in relation to food, eating, and body image.

In the context of BED, CBT is meticulously tailored to help individuals gain insight into the links between their thoughts, emotions, and binge eating episodes. It's an empowering process where one learns to identify and challenge distorted beliefs that perpetuate the cycle of binging, such as "all-or-nothing" thinking or self-critical paradigms about weight and self-worth. Therapists guide patients in the development of strategies to reshape these beliefs and manage the impulses that lead to binge eating, often using tangible tools such as food diaries and situational analysis to bring the abstract into concrete focus.

What sets CBT apart is its action-oriented approach. Patients are not only encouraged to talk about their struggles but are also actively engaged in practicing new habits on a daily basis. This might involve setting realistic goals, improving problem-solving skills, and experimenting with new ways to cope with emotions and stress that don't involve food. The emphasis here is on incremental change, which not only facilitates improvement in eating behaviors but also engenders broader improvements in patients' mental health and overall quality of life.

It is important to address the empirical support that underscores CBT's prowess in the realm of BED. Research consistently shows that CBT results in a significant reduction in binge eating frequency, with a noteworthy proportion of individuals achieving abstinence from binge eating post-treatment. More impressively, these improvements are largely maintained at long-term follow-up, highlighting the durable impact of the CBT intervention. This durability is critical, as BED is not only disruptive in the short term but can also have far-reaching implications if left unaddressed.

By actively engaging in this therapeutic process, individuals not only work towards eradicating symptoms but also embark on a transformative journey to reclaim control over their lives.

Interpersonal Psychotherapy (IPT)

is a therapeutic approach that has shown considerable promise in addressing the underlying interpersonal issues that often coexist with Binge Eating Disorder (BED). Emerging from the understanding that the quality of our relationships can significantly influence our eating behaviors, IPT posits that by improving interpersonal functioning, individuals can achieve more control over their eating patterns.

Unlike therapies that focus solely on the individual's thoughts or behaviors, IPT works by exploring the client's social context and targeting interpersonal problems, which may trigger or exacerbate episodes of binge eating. In the core of IPT lies the theory that once a person improves how they communicate and navigate social roles, they gain emotional support and stress-relieving outlets that diminish the need to turn to food for comfort.

Implementing IPT involves several stages, beginning with an initial assessment where the therapist and client identify key interpersonal issues. These commonly include unresolved grief, role disputes or transitions, and interpersonal deficits. After identification, the therapist helps the client to develop strategies for tackling these problems, thus removing or alleviating interpersonal triggers for binge eating behaviors. In the midst of these challenges, the motivational nature of IPT encourages clients to become active agents in their recovery, engendering a sense of hope and the confidence needed to effect meaningful change.

Studies have shown that IPT can be as effective as Cognitive-Behavioral Therapy (CBT) for BED, particularly in maintaining long-term results. Importantly, IPT addresses the social deficits and supports the development of healthier relationships, which can sustain recovery and enhance overall well-being. As such, IPT might not only serve as a direct intervention for binge eating but also as a preventive measure against relapse by fortifying the client's interpersonal resilience.

The book's exploration of IPT as a treatment for BED intertwines scientific research with an understanding of the human story behind each case of BED. This holistic perspective illuminates the pathway to recovery that exists when personal agency is coupled with evidence-based interventions, like IPT, to address the complexity of factors contributing to binge eating. In the continuation of this book, the focus will remain on such integrated strategies and how they can initiate a journey toward healing and long-term wellness.

Medication and Pharmacotherapy

As individuals grappling with binge eating disorder (BED) continue to seek effective treatments, medication and pharmacotherapy emerge as vital components in the arsenal against this relentless condition. In the context of BED, pharmaceutical intervention can be a beacon of hope for those who have found therapy and lifestyle changes alone to be insufficient. This section delves into the medications approved for BED treatment and how they function to alleviate symptoms, while acknowledging pharmacotherapy as an adjunct to comprehensive treatment strategies.

Pharmacotherapy for BED primarily aims to regulate neurotransmitters involved in appetite control and mood. Selective serotonin reuptake inhibitors (SSRIs) have been studied in the treatment of BED with varying degrees of success; they work by increasing serotonin levels in the brain, which can help reduce the frequency of binge eating episodes. For instance, fluoxetine (Prozac), an SSRI, is approved by the FDA for the treatment of depression and has been used off-label to address BED.

Another class of drugs that has shown promise is the stimulants, particularly those approved for attention deficit hyperactivity disorder (ADHD). Lisdexamfetamine (Vyvanse) is the first drug explicitly approved by the FDA specifically for the treatment of moderate to severe BED in adults. It acts by increasing levels of dopamine and norepinephrine, thereby improving impulse control and reducing the focus on food.

While these medications show potential, it is imperative to understand that they aren't a catch-all solution. Each individual with BED has a unique set of biological, psychological, and environmental factors contributing to their condition. Hence, medication may work optimally when combined with psychotherapy, nutritional support, and lifestyle modifications to tackle those multifaceted needs.

One must consider the side effects that accompany the use of pharmacotherapy in treating BED. SSRIs can bring about sexual dysfunction, nausea, or insomnia, while stimulants may lead to increased heart rate, insomnia, or anxiety. These adverse effects call for a cautious approach; clinicians must weigh the benefits of medication against the risks, tailoring treatments to the individual's situation and monitoring response and tolerance closely.

For those contemplating pharmacotherapy, a comprehensive evaluation by a healthcare professional specialized in eating disorders is a critical first step. A personalized treatment plan will likely incorporate a thorough medical examination to rule out physiological contributors to binge eating, a discussion of treatment history, and psychological assessment to address co-occurring mental health conditions.

Relapse is always a concern with BED, as with other psychiatric conditions. Medication can play a part in relapse prevention by stabilizing mood fluctuations and controlling impulses long-term, thus helping individuals stay on the path to recovery. However, it is also essential to establish appropriate exit strategies for medication, including tapering doses to avoid withdrawal symptoms while ensuring continuous support through therapy and coping strategies are in place.

In conclusion, while pharmacotherapy offers significant benefits and can be part of a comprehensive treatment approach for BED, it is not a standalone cure. The roadmap to recovery involves a combination of medication, counseling, and support, meticulously crafted to each person's journey. As the research evolves, new pharmacological options may emerge, providing additional hope and assistance in the relentless fight against the cycles of binge eating.

Chapter 10:
Beyond the Individual: The Role of Community and Society

The journey to understanding and managing Binge Eating Disorder (BED) doesn't end with individual efforts; it's a path that weaves through the heart of our communities and the broader fabric of society. While Chapters 1 through 9 equipped us with knowledge about BED, its diagnosis, implications, and treatments, Chapter 10 ventures into the collective role that community and society play in the healing process. The presence of a supportive community, along with sweeping societal changes, can create an environment where individuals battling BED can thrive. Encouragement can be found in communal groups fostering connection and understanding that no one needs to face their challenges alone. Advocacy within societal structures facilitates the development of policies that ensure access to appropriate care and the dismantling of harmful beauty standards that contribute to the disorder's prevalence. As we explore the transformative potential of community initiatives and societal reforms, we lay the groundwork for not only individual recovery but also a global sea change in addressing the complexities of BED.

Community Support and Groups

As we pivot from individual management strategies to the broader context of recovery, one cannot underestimate the power of community support and groups in the journey toward healing. Amidst battling Binge Eating Disorder (BED), the comfort derived from connecting with those who truly understand cannot be overstated. Community support, be it in the form of online forums, local support groups, or structured therapy groups, offers a refuge where shared experiences and collective wisdom pave the road to recovery (Miller & Willer, 2023).

Possessing a non-judgmental space where vulnerabilities can be voiced and accomplishments celebrated is a cornerstone of lasting change. Research has consistently highlighted the efficacy of group therapy, particularly when combining psychoeducation with peer support, in enhancing treatment outcomes for individuals with BED (Thompson et al., 2022). Not only does it reduce the sense of isolation, but it also fosters accountability and provides practical coping strategies that are often born from the lived expertise within the group. Therefore, seeking out and joining community support should be considered a pivotal element in one's treatment plan, as it complements the efforts made in more formal therapeutic settings and fortifies one's resolve to persist through the challenges of overcoming BED.

Additionally, support groups often serve as a gateway to a broader community involvement, where advocacy and collective action can lead to societal changes. This engagement further empowers individuals by providing a sense of purpose and belonging that extends beyond their personal struggles. It's a dynamic symbiosis; as individuals draw strength from the community, they, in turn, contribute to the community's resilience and capacity to support others in similar plights (Jenkins & Kendler, 2023). To neglect the potential of community support is to overlook a vital resource in the multi-faceted approach required to address BED effectively.

Advocacy and Policy Change

As we delve deeper into the implications and necessary interventions for overcoming Binge Eating Disorder (BED), it becomes increasingly clear that individual efforts, while essential, can only go so far without broader societal support. Advocacy and policy change represent pivotal arenas where concerted efforts can lead to meaningful progress in the fight against BED. The influence of legislation, healthcare policies, and public health initiatives can shape the accessibility and quality of services for those grappling with BED, as well as influence the larger societal understanding of this disorder.

Advocating for policy change demands a multifaceted approach, calling for collaborations between individuals, healthcare professionals, and lawmakers. Changing the landscape of mental health policy involves not only raising awareness about BED but also convincing policymakers of the importance of including it in healthcare coverage and funding research. A growing body of scientific evidence supports the classification of BED as a significant public health issue (Brownley et al., 2016). This research is critical when advocating for the development of comprehensive treatment programs, insurance coverage, and the establishment of standardized care protocols.

Moreover, the call to advocacy transcends healthcare policy. It must also address societal norms that inadvertently perpetuate harmful stereotypes regarding body image and eating behaviors. Advocates play a vital role in challenging these norms by promoting body positivity and educating the public about the complexity of eating disorders. Changes in policy can encourage media representation that aligns more closely with the diversity of body types and experiences, rather than perpetuating unrealistic beauty standards.

Challenging Societal Norms and Beauty Standards

In the voyage towards understanding and managing Binge Eating Disorder (BED), it is essential to confront the omnipresent societal norms and beauty standards that often play a silent but potent role in the lives of individuals affected by this disorder. Beauty standards, perpetuated through media and cultural norms, can contribute to the deep-seated feelings of inadequacy and low self-esteem that fuel disordered eating behaviors.

The incessant barrage of images showcasing idealized bodies and lifestyles can lead to a relentless pursuit of thinness or a particular appearance, which can be detrimental to one's mental health. The perceived need to conform to these standards can exacerbate feelings of isolation and shame, which are common among individuals with BED. It is confrontational, yet necessary, to question and redefine what is considered beautiful or desirable within our society.

Addressing these societal pressures begins with fostering awareness of the diverse types of beauty that exist beyond the narrow confines of current standards. Encouraging the representation of a wide range of body sizes, shapes, and appearances in the media can help lessen the stigma around bodies that don't fit the conventional mold. People with BED benefit from understanding that self-worth is not contingent upon meeting these often unachievable standards.

Beyond the individual, there is a growing movement aimed at changing the narrative surrounding body image. Campaigns that highlight body positivity and inclusiveness are crucial in this regard. Beauty is being redefined in more holistic terms, emphasizing health and well-being over appearance. This movement not only offers comfort but also empowers those grappling with BED to challenge the status quo and embrace their unique selves.

In the therapeutic setting, helping individuals with BED to develop resilience against societal pressures is paramount. Therapies like Cognitive-Behavioral Therapy (CBT) can assist patients in recognizing and altering negative thought patterns about their bodies and self-worth. Moreover, support groups and community initiatives provide a platform for sharing experiences and reinforcing the idea that one's value is not dependent on their physical attributes.

It is essential to recognize that changing entrenched societal norms is a process that requires the collective effort of individuals, health professionals, media, and policymakers. Advocacy for more inclusive health and beauty standards can play a pivotal role in this transformation. Education campaigns targeted at youths can preempt the internalization of harmful standards by instilling confidence and body acceptance from an early age.

In light of addressing BED, we must also challenge the diet culture that pervades much of society, promoting an often unhealthy and obsessive focus on weight loss rather than on overall health and well-being. The endorsement of body diversity and the decoupling of self-esteem from body size are steps towards dismantling the harmful effects of diet culture.

All these efforts contribute to the broader societal change, which is not merely beneficial for those with BED but also for the population at large. A society that welcomes and celebrates diversity in body shape and size breeds an environment where fewer individuals feel pressured to conform through harmful means, including binge eating as a coping mechanism.

The conversation on challenging societal norms and beauty standards is not merely academic. It is a clarion call for change, a necessary step in the holistic treatment and management of BED, and the cultivation of a society that upholds the health and well-being of its members above unrealistic aesthetic ideals.

Chapter 11:
Long-term Recovery and Relapse Prevention

In the ongoing journey toward healing from Binge Eating Disorder, sustaining the hard-won progress beyond the immediate treatment phase is both challenging and critical. Long-term recovery is not merely the absence of symptoms; it is the continual cultivation of a balanced relationship with food and oneself. It encompasses the vigilant maintenance of healthy habits, a sound support system, and adaptive coping mechanisms that together create a safety net against relapse. Relapse prevention is a multifaceted endeavor that involves monitoring for warning signs, implementing strategies for managing stressors, and staying connected with therapeutic resources. According to the research, structured relapse prevention programs can significantly reduce the frequency and severity of relapses. Such programs, coupled with ongoing support, empower individuals to navigate the complexities of recovery with confidence and resilience. It's essential to recognize that setbacks are a natural part of the recovery process, not a failure, and each challenge faced is an opportunity to reinforce one's commitment to health. Recovery from BED isn't a linear path but rather a lifelong journey of self-discovery and growth, where each day brings us closer to a harmonious existence.

Setting Realistic Goals and Expectations

Embarking on the path to recovery from Binge Eating Disorder (BED) necessitates a compassionate yet strategic mindset, beginning with the establishment of realistic goals and expectations. It's essential for individuals to understand that progress is incremental and subject to each person's unique context, including their health status, personal circumstances, and resources available. Unrealistic aspirations of rapid transformation or perfection may precipitate frustration and self-criticism, undermining the very foundation of recovery. Thus, goals ought to be tailored to achievable milestones that encourage a sense of accomplishment and propel the individual toward recovery with consistency and patience.

Goal setting in the context of overcoming BED often involves behavioral changes, such as establishing regular meal patterns or learning healthier coping mechanisms for stress (Wonderlich et al., 2020). These objectives should be clear and measurable and might include time-oriented targets to help track progress and adjust strategies as necessary. Importantly, while treatment effectiveness is a critical component of goal setting, it's also vital to have adaptive goals that center on the individual's well-being rather than solely on eliminating binging symptoms. This holistic approach emphasizes recovery as a broader enhancement of life's quality rather than a singular focus on eating behaviors.

It's crucial to acknowledge the role of patience and self-compassion within the goal-setting framework. However, these setbacks are not failures but opportunities to learn and refine coping strategies. Individuals are encouraged to celebrate small victories and to consider setbacks as part of the journey, realigning their strategies and maintaining their commitment to recovery rather than feeling defeated. Fostering resilience through adaptable expectations helps in sustaining long-term efforts toward wellness.

Clear communication regarding achievable goals can facilitate a supportive environment conducive to recovery. Educating stakeholders about BED, its challenges, and recovery can foster empathy and strengthen the support system necessary for the individual's journey.

As recovery unfolds, recalibrating goals and expectations to align with personal growth and changing circumstances is an ongoing process, integral to fostering a sustainable, healthier relationship with food and oneself.

Strategies for Sustaining Progress

In our journey through the complexities of Binge Eating Disorder (BED), we've traversed a myriad of terrains—from understanding its very nature to confronting its psychological underpinnings and physiological impacts. As we delve into maintaining the momentum of recovery, it's paramount that the strategies we adopt are not just effective, but sustainable. Sustained progress in combating BED requires a robust framework that braces one for the long haul, keeping relapses at bay and empowerment at the forefront.

Sustainability begins with the acknowledgment that recovery is non-linear. Crafting a personal toolkit of strategies bolstered by both resolve and flexibility sets a foundation for enduring success. Prioritizing self-compassion is one such cornerstone. Studies show that lessening self-criticism and embracing kindness towards oneself can significantly bolster recovery from eating disorders.

Establishing strong routines is another pivotal strategy. Routines erect a framework around which daily life is structured, offering stability in times of tumult. This might include regular meal planning—a technique already identified as conducive to managing BED.

Continuing therapy, whether it's cognitive-behavioral therapy (CBT), interpersonal psychotherapy (IPT), or another modality, is crucial for sustaining progress. Therapy provides ongoing support, helping to navigate the emotional triggers and stressors that could lead to recurrence.

Staying connected with support systems—be they professional counselors, support groups, or loved ones—serves as a lifeline. Sustaining progress in combatting BED isn't solitary; it's a collective endeavor. The input and understanding from others can provide perspective, encouragement, and wisdom, especially during challenging episodes.

Another strategy is continuous learning and self-awareness. Keeping abreast of new findings related to BED can inform one's approach to recovery and provide access to alternative therapies and tools. This might involve engaging in workshops, reading current literature on the subject, and being open to adjusting one's treatment plan in response to new evidence.

Finally, setting achievable, measurable goals can reinforce one's sense of progress and provide clear milestones that fuel motivation. This entails both short-term objectives for the immediate future, as well as longer-term aspirations that provide a sense of direction and purpose.

Dealing with Setbacks

Managing BED is not simply about eradicating the disorder entirely from the first attempt; it's about learning to navigate through the relapses and using them as stepping stones for long-term success. This chapter is dedicated to understanding how to handle those moments when you feel like you have regressed and how to turn them into opportunities for growth.

Building resilience against triggers is another crucial aspect. Identifying what prompts the recurrence of binge eating behaviors and developing a toolkit of coping strategies can provide a sense of control and readiness.

Moreover, reassessing and adjusting your recovery goals may be necessary after a setback. Goals should be SMART: Specific, Measurable, Attainable, Relevant, and Time-bound. Sometimes, setbacks can occur because previous goals were too ambitious or vague, so recalibrating them to be more achievable can prevent future disappointments.

Throughout this process, professional help can be invaluable. Therapy sessions provide a safe environment to explore what went wrong and why. A therapist can offer guidance on coping strategies and might suggest adjustments in treatment like medication or different therapeutic approaches if necessary.

Chapter 12:
The Future of BED Research and Treatments

In this momentous chapter, we set our sights toward a horizon teeming with promise and new discoveries—the ever-evolving field of Binge Eating Disorder (BED) research and the treatments that await. The ongoing pursuit of knowledge has myriad scientists and doctors at the precipice of breakthroughs that could forever alter the landscape of BED treatment. Imagine a world where the enigmatic genetic markers of BED are not only understood but can be influenced to prevent or mitigate the compulsion to binge. Innovations in technology offer unprecedented tools, from apps that provide instant therapeutic support to wearable devices monitoring physiological indicators of stress, possibly predicting and intervening before a binge occurs. Progress in the realm of epigenetics hints at a future where the environment's role in shaping gene expression becomes an integral part of personalized therapy plans. As we stand on the cusp of these advancements, we are called to foster an environment of optimism, ensuring that those grappling with BED have access to the leading edge of therapeutic interventions and are welcomed into an era defined by revolutionary care and understanding.

Emerging Therapies

In a landscape ever-evolving with scientific discovery, new and innovative treatments for Binge Eating Disorder (BED) are on the horizon. These emergent therapies aim to address the complexities of BED with greater precision and personalization than ever before. They hold the potential not only to treat but to revolutionize the understanding and management of this condition, offering a beacon of hope to those entrenched in the cycle of binge eating.

One such therapy that has garnered attention is neuromodulation, particularly transcranial magnetic stimulation (TMS). This non-invasive technique uses magnetic fields to stimulate nerve cells in specific areas of the brain associated with impulse control and mood regulation. Early studies suggest that TMS may help reduce binge eating episodes and improve executive function for individuals with BED (Dunner et al., 2022). As TMS therapy becomes more refined, it could become a cornerstone in managing BED by targeting the neurological underpinnings directly.

Another emerging therapy is the use of virtual reality (VR). Though it may seem like the stuff of science fiction, VR has made its way into psychological treatments, providing immersive environments where individuals can confront and work through their triggers in a controlled setting. By simulating real-life scenarios, VR can offer a unique and impactful form of exposure therapy, helping to reduce anxiety and binge eating behaviors in a safe space before transitioning those coping skills to the real world (Ferrer-García & Gutiérrez-Maldonado, 2022).

On the biochemical front, new medications are also under trial, aiming to go beyond the typical appetite suppressants and antidepressants. These novel pharmacological agents target specific neurotransmitters and hormones implicated in hunger and satiety signaling pathways. The development of such medications seeks not just to curb the urge to binge but to correct the underlying biochemical dysregulation that contributes to BED (Bello & Yeomans, 2023).

Lastly, integrated therapeutic approaches combining cognitive-behavioral principles with nutritional guidance, mindfulness practices, and personalized medicine are gaining traction. These multifaceted programs are designed to address all aspects of BED—biological, psychological, and social—allowing for a more holistic and enduring recovery. As research burgeons in this domain, it inspires a more comprehensive and compassionate approach to treatment, tailoring interventions to the unique profile of each individual (Smith & Robbins, 2023).

These emerging therapies reflect the innovative spirit driving the future of BED treatment. They underscore a commitment to understanding and addressing this disorder with the nuance it requires, based on the latest scientific evidence. As individuals and professionals continue to advocate for advanced research and better access to treatment, there is a mounting sense of optimism that the fight against BED will be met with ever more effective weapons in the arsenal of mental health care.

Technological Advancements

In the frontier of battling Binge Eating Disorder (BED), technology has emerged as a powerful ally. As we navigate the complexities of BED, it's important to highlight the innovative tools and methods that are transforming the way we understand, treat, and manage this disorder. Technological advancements are revolutionizing patient care, providing unprecedented opportunities for diagnosis, treatment personalization, and patient empowerment.

The introduction of mobile health applications has created new possibilities for individuals with BED to monitor their eating habits, mood fluctuations, and triggers in real-time (Munsch et al., 2021). These applications often incorporate elements of Cognitive-Behavioral Therapy (CBT) and self-monitoring techniques, enabling users to identify patterns and intervene before a binge occurs. They're not just passive trackers – many are interactive, offering coping strategies and mindfulness exercises, bridging the gap between therapy sessions and daily life. The implementation of teletherapy platforms has also expanded accessibility, allowing individuals to receive professional support from the comfort of their own homes, thus overcoming barriers related to geography, mobility, or stigma.

Advancements in neuroimaging technology have shed light on the neural underpinnings of BED. Sophisticated techniques like functional magnetic resonance imaging (fMRI) allow researchers to observe brain activity in response to food stimuli and emotional provocations (Schienle et al., 2018). These insights contribute to a more nuanced understanding of the disorder and inform the development of targeted intervention strategies. By identifying the neural circuits that may predispose someone to binge eating, interventions can be tailored to modify these specific pathways, potentially enhancing treatment outcomes.

Another promising frontier is the use of virtual reality (VR) in exposure therapy for BED. VR provides a safe and controlled environment where individuals can confront and learn to manage their cravings without the risk of actual bingeing (Ferrer-Garcia et al., 2017). This immersive technology facilitates the simulation of real-world scenarios, offering a practical means of practicing coping strategies and strengthening self-regulation skills. The potential for VR in the treatment of BED is immense, as it holds the capability to simulate trigger situations, foster healthier decision-making, and ultimately change behavioral responses to food cues.

Yet, it's crucial to approach these technological innovations with a balanced perspective. While they offer promising adjuncts to traditional treatments, personal touch and professional guidance remain irreplaceable components of effective BED management. A synergistic blend of technology and human expertise will likely define the future of BED treatment. For those struggling with this disorder, the advent of technology brings hope – the hope of more personalized care, greater access to resources, and ultimately, a firmer grasp on recovery.

The Horizon of Genetic and Epigenetic Research

In our quest to understand the intricacies of Binge Eating Disorder (BED), we stand on the precipice of a new and thrilling epoch in scientific discovery. Genetic and epigenetic research offers unparalleled opportunities to unravel the biological components that contribute to this complex disorder. By digging into the bedrock of our very essence—our DNA—we open up avenues for personalized treatments and interventions that could transform the lives of those grappling with BED.

The examination of genetic factors revolves around identifying specific gene variations that may predispose an individual to develop BED. Various studies have begun to spotlight certain genes that are more prevalent amongst those with eating disorders, including BED (Trace et al., 2013). These genetic markers may one day serve as beacons, guiding us towards early detection and prevention strategies. Our DNA does not act in isolation; rather, it is in constant interplay with environmental influences, and this is where epigenetics comes to the forefront.

Epigenetics, a field of study looking beyond the genetic sequence, investigates how external factors can switch genes on or off without altering the underlying DNA sequence. Epigenetic modifications, triggered by experiences such as stress or trauma, might explain why some individuals with a genetic vulnerability to BED end up manifesting the disorder while others do not (Mehler et al., 2018). These insights are crucial; they emphasize that our genes are not our destiny, and that the environment we inhabit plays a pivotal role in our health outcomes.

Moreover, research into the epigenetic mechanisms of BED suggests that interventions might not only target the disorder's symptoms but could potentially reverse the epigenetic changes themselves (Booij et al., 2016). This means we could eventually recalibrate the biological underpinnings that contribute to the disorder, effectively 'rewiring' the body's response to triggers and challenges that precipitate binge eating.

As we edge closer to understanding the genetic and epigenetic landscape of BED, we must also grapple with the ethical implications. The possibility of genetic screening for BED raises questions about privacy, discrimination, and the psychological impact of knowing one's genetic risk. It's imperative that as we push forward in our scientific pursuit, we do so with a framework that respects individual rights and promotes equitable access to any emerging interventions.

One of the most promising aspects of genetic and epigenetic research is its potential to tailor treatments to the individual. Instead of the 'one-size-fits-all' approach, we can foresee a future where therapies are customized based on a person's unique genetic makeup. This precision medicine could lead to more effective outcomes, as treatments dovetail with the individual characteristics of each person's disorder (Bulik et al., 2016).

Meanwhile, for those currently on the journey towards recovery, the promise of genetic and epigenetic research offers hope. Hope that their struggle is seen and understood on the most fundamental level, and that the solutions of tomorrow may lie within the very blueprint of their being. As research unfolds, it also becomes a beacon of education, teaching us that BED is not a choice, but a disorder influenced by a complex interplay of genetic and environmental factors.

We stand at the dawn of this new era with cautious optimism. The horizon gleams with potential breakthroughs that may shift the paradigm of how we approach BED. However, we must continue to move forward mindfully, acknowledging the tremendous responsibility that comes with unlocking the secrets coded within us. With perseverance and ethical vigilance, the horizon of genetic and epigenetic research could lead to an age of understanding and healing that once seemed beyond our grasp.

As we continue to chart the course of BED research, it's essential to remain focused on the individuals behind the data—human beings searching for relief and healing. Their stories and experiences must guide our scientific exploration and remind us why the pursuit of this knowledge is not merely academic, but a deeply human endeavor aimed at alleviating suffering and improving quality of life.

Conclusion

In the preceding chapters, we have journeyed through the intricate landscape of Binge Eating Disorder (BED), unraveling its complexities and investigating the myriad of ways it can be addressed and, ultimately, overcome. Standing now at the culmination of our exploration, we find ourselves armed with knowledge—equipped not only to identify and understand BED but empowered to embark on a transformative path toward recovery. Knowledge, alongside compassion and tenacity, becomes our beacon, guiding us through the challenges and setbacks that are inherent in confronting this pervasive disorder (Wilfley et al., 2020).

Embracing this newfound understanding, one must acknowledge the power of individual agency in the healing process. While BED is undeniably intertwined with biological, psychological, and social variables, the heart of this journey lies within the self. Emphasizing self-compassion and resilience, it is essential to utilize the tools and strategies discussed—from medical interventions and therapy approaches to lifestyle adjustments and community support. Remember, every step taken is a step towards a future where BED no longer defines one's life; a future brimming with health, self-mastery, and fulfillment.

In closing, confronting BED is not a journey one must walk alone. In the veil of darkness that BED casts, let this book serve as a lighthouse, providing direction and assurance. Be encouraged to step forward with courage, drawing on the collective wisdom and empathy of those who walk with you—clinicians, researchers, loved ones, and fellow travelers on this path. Seek out your support, honor your progress, however incremental, and believe in the possibility of a restored and balanced relationship with food and yourself. Let the knowledge you've gained be your steadfast companion as you reclaim control, rediscover joy, and reshape your story. As you close this book, open the chapter of your life where BED is but a footnote to your triumphant narrative (Grilo, 2017).

Appendix A:
Appendix

The journey through understanding and combating Binge Eating Disorder (BED) has been a complex tapestry woven with threads of psychological insight, physiological knowledge, and the determination for transformation. As we close this book, it's crucial to have a compass that points towards the path ahead. Appendix A is that compass—comprised of curated resources, a selected bibliography for further reading that deepens your understanding, and practical checklists and worksheets that translate knowledge into action.

Resources and Support Networks

In your quest for guidance and communal support, there are beacons of hope and solidarity. Community organizations, helplines, and online forums can offer a hand to hold when the path feels solitary. Reaching out is not a testament to weakness, but an act of bravery. The National Eating Disorders Association (NEDA) is a cornerstone where you can begin, with connections to support groups, education, and a helpline to directly address your concerns (NEDA, 2022).

Checklists and Worksheets

Applying theoretical knowledge to everyday living is a monumental step. Accessible checklists and worksheets empower you to identify triggers, plan meals, and monitor progress.

Remember that the real story is not solely in the unmasking of the disorder but in the relentless pursuit of healing and the courage to face each day anew. May this appendix serve not as the final word, but as an anchoring section, reminding us that the journey towards health is ongoing, and that the tools and support you need are within reach.

Resources and Support Networks

In charting a path through the complexities of Binge Eating Disorder (BED), the importance of resources and support networks can't be overstated. Availing oneself of a robust support network is tantamount to equipping oneself with an arsenal to combat the battles that lie within. As individuals grappling with BED begin to peel back the layers of their eating habits, identifying the support systems available becomes crucial to recovery. Many will find solace in peer support groups, which provide not only a haven for shared experiences but also a sense of belonging that can fortify one's resolve in facing BED (Hartmann et al., 2012). The BED community is replete with specialized support groups, both in-person and online, which serve as communal touchstones where one can engage with others on a similar journey, fostering an environment of mutual understanding and continuous support.

Professional resources such as counseling services, dietitians specialized in eating disorders, and medical professionals should also be integral components of an individual's support framework. It's essential to cultivate a multidisciplinary team that comprehends the multifaceted nature of BED. This team approach not only ensures a comprehensive treatment plan but also envelops the individual in an interconnected web of care. Moreover, several non-profit organizations provide educational materials, workshops, and seminars aimed at expanding knowledge, reducing stigma, and empowering those with BED to understand and manage their condition effectively.

As fundamental as it is to recognize the available resources, it is equally critical for individuals to nurture their personal support networks. Friends, family members, and loved ones play a pivotal role in providing emotional sustenance.

www.ingramcontent.com/pod-product-compliance
Lightning Source LLC
Chambersburg PA
CBHW020338290526
45785CB00005B/2082